# HYPNOSIS FOR WEIGHT LOSS:

STOP COMPULSIVE EATING AND SUGAR CRAVING, REACH HEALTHY HABITS, UNLOCK YOUR MIND WITH POSITIVE AFFIRMATIONS, FILL YOUR LIFE WITH SELF-LOVE. EAT LESS WITH HYPNOTIC GASTRIC BAND

**ERIKA YOUNG**

# TABLE OF CONTENTS

# Introduction

Hypnosis for weight loss is basically using hypnosis techniques to allow you to lose weight. It's a way to shed a few extra pounds. But most of the time, it is paired with a diet plan. It is advisable that you continue a good regimen of food, followed by moderate exercise. But this will allow you to lose weight faster, and if you're a person who has cravings for things, then this will help you immensely.

It's also a part of the counseling that some people get. You'll be able to get help on your issues regarding food, and this form of hypnosis will allow you to have a better time with your cravings. You can do this with a professional, but you can also do it on your own. It'll allow you to be in control of your life, and you'll control those bad cravings you have.

How it works is simple. When you're using hypnosis, you're in a state of absorption and concentration. You're also in a very relaxed and suggestible state, so whatever is said to you is basically taken in a literal manner. You will use mental images to convey the meaning of the words that are said. You'll have your attention focused on that, and when your mind is in a state of concentration, you'll start to have your subconscious handle your cravings. It's a remarkable way to keep yourself in check, and you'll be able to lose a few extra pounds while still trying to keep your body in shape. It's best if you do this with a diet and exercise routine, for it'll allow you to get through it better and achieve more results.

It's best to do this when you have a window of time ready for you to take care of this issue. You'll want at least thirty minutes of quiet time to handle these cravings, ideally an hour at most. You will be handling some pretty heavy matters, so making sure that you're relaxed and able to come back to reality before and after the hypnosis will make it all the better.

The effectiveness varies from person to person. It will help you, and, on average, a person loses about six pounds. You might lose more, but you might not lose as much as expected. If you're trying to lose a ton of weight, this might not help. But, if you're looking to help eliminate cravings in your life and live a healthier lifestyle, then this is definitely the right tool for you. It's a way to help you supplement your exercising plans, and with this, you'll be able to have an even better time when it comes to shedding those pounds fast.

There are other benefits of using hypnosis for weight loss. The obvious big one is that you lose weight. That's the one people will notice. You'll start to shed those pounds, and you might lose more than you expected. It won't be significant, such as like fifty pounds or more, but if you want to help your body and allow yourself the benefits of being able to control the cravings to lose weight, then this is perfect for you. Another benefit that people don't realize is how relaxed you are. You'll actually be able to become more relaxed as a result of this. By relaxing the body, you'll be able to also reduce your blood pressure levels and even stop the risk of heart disease. Hypnosis for weight loss allows you to put yourself in a relaxed state for at least an hour, and when you wake up, you'll feel more relaxed. It can also help with bodily tissues, such as muscle aches and pains. If you want to use this to help with those issues as well, it'll definitely do the trick.

Then there are the lasting benefits of it. These are the benefits that you'll get because of the hypnosis. When you're doing this, you'll be able to tackle those parts of your subconscious that think it's okay to eat when you're stressed, or it'll tell you to eat more than necessary. Sometimes, your mind can be your own worst enemy, and this is certainly one of those times. With hypnosis for weight loss, you'll allow yourself to handle your body in a positive manner. If you do this, you'll actually allow yourself to control your cravings and desires through the use of hypnosis. It might seem crazy, but it is possible. It's a great way to take life by the horns, and by doing this, you'll be able to allow yourself the benefit of controlling the factors in your life, such as stress or how much you eat, and turning them around to give yourself a more positive image that will benefit you in ways you've never expected before.

If you're the type of person who wants to change your life and your way of thinking to live a healthier life, then hypnosis for weight loss is perfect for you. With this technique, you'll be targeting different parts of the body, and by doing this, you'll be able to have a much better time when it comes to getting rid of the excess weight. It's a great way to lose weight, and by the end of it, you'll be happier, and the scale will look like a friend, instead of an enemy.

# 1. Psychology of Hypnosis

## Hypnosis in Psychology

While definitions may contrast, the American Psychological Association characterizes hypnosis as an agreeable collaboration in which the member responds to the hypnotist's recommendations. Because of basic acts, the trance has turned out to be notable where people are urged to direct unprecedented or silly conduct, yet also clinically demonstrated to give medicinal and restorative favorable circumstances, mosquitoes. Hypnosis has even been recommended to diminish dementia manifestations.

What do you think when you hear the term trance specialist? In case you're similar to numerous people, the term may invoke photos of a vile stage miscreant who, by swinging a pocket watch to and fro, makes a sleep-inducing state.

Truth be told, there is little similitude among mesmerizing and these cliché portrayals. "The trance specialist doesn't mesmerize the person, as indicated by analyst John Kihlstrom. Or maybe, the trance specialist fills in as a sort of mentor or coach whose assignment is to help the individual turned out to be mesmerized."

While hypnosis, or even, spellbinding is regularly characterized as a rest, like a dazed state, it is better explained as a condition of concentrated consideration, expanded suggestive and clear dreams. Individuals in a mesmerized state frequently appear to be lethargic and daydreaming, yet they are in a condition of hyper-cognizance truth be told.

Spellbinding is now and then alluded to as hypnotherapy in brain research and has been utilized for a few reasons, including agony abatement and treatment. Ordinarily, trance is finished by a certified specialist who uses perception and verbal reiteration to cause an entrancing condition.

## Impacts of Hypnosis

Entrancing knowledge can vary significantly from individual to person. Some spellbound individuals report feeling separation or outrageous unwinding during the mesmerizing state while others even think their exercises have all the earmarks of being occurring outside their cognizant will. Other individuals, while under spellbinding, may remain completely cognizant and ready to lead talks.

Scientist Ernest Hilgard's examinations demonstrated how spellbinding could be utilized to drastically change discernments. The member's arm was then placed in ice water in the wake of training a mesmerized individual not to feel torment in their arm while individuals who were not spellbound needed to expel their arm from the water.

## Where is Hypnotism Utilized?

Through research, spellbinding has been utilized in the treatment of different conditions, for example,

- Alleviating constant excruciating conditions like rheumatoid joint pain
- Alleviating and treating torment in labor
- Reducing dementia side effects
- For some ADHD side effects, hypnotherapy might be of assistance
- Reducing the impacts of sickness prompting retching in disease patients on chemotherapy
- Reducing torment when experiencing a dental technique

- Improving and taking out skin conditions, for example, psoriasis and moles
- Reducing touchy inside disorder manifestations

So, for what reason should an individual endeavor in spellbinding? In certain examples, people might search for entrancing to help constant agony or ease torment and nervousness brought about by restorative procedures, for example, medical procedure or birth.

Mesmerizing has likewise been utilized to help people with conduct changes, for example, smoking end, weight reduction, or bed-wetting counteractive action.

## Is it possible to hypnotize yourself?

While numerous people accept that they can't be hypnotized, a study has demonstrated that numerous individuals are more hypnotizable than they might suspect.

- Fifteen percent of people are profoundly receptive to spellbinding.
- Children are bound to be inclined to spellbinding.
- It is respected hard or difficult to spellbind around 10% of grown-ups.
- People who can ingest themselves promptly in dreams are substantially more receptive to spellbinding.

If you are keen on being mesmerized, moving toward the involvement with a receptive outlook is basic to recall. Research has proposed that individuals who take a good viewpoint of mesmerizing will, in general, respond better.

## Theories on Hypnosis

Extraordinary compared to other realized hypotheses is Hilgard's mesmerizing hypothesis of neo-dissociation.5 According to Hilgard, people in an entrancing state experience an isolated cognizance wherein two unmistakable surges of mental movement are available.

While one continuous flow responds to the recommendations of the subliminal specialist, another flood of separated information system outside the cognizant familiarity with the entranced person.

## Myths about Hypnosis

It is common to misjudge the topic of hypnotism. That is why myths and half-truths abound about this matter.

Myth: You won't recall that anything that happened when you were mesmerized when you wake up from a trance.

While amnesia may occur in uncommon cases, during mesmerizing, people more often than not recollect everything that unfolded. Mesmerizing, be that as it may, can have a significant memory impact. Posthypnotic amnesia may make an individual overlook a portion of the stuff that occurred previously or during spellbinding. This effect, be that as it may, is typically confined and impermanent.

Myth: Hypnosis can help people to recall the exact date of wrongdoing they have been seeing.

While spellbinding can be utilized to improve memory, the effects in well-known media have been significantly misrepresented. Research has discovered that trance doesn't bring about noteworthy memory improvement or precision, and entrancing may, in reality, lead to false or misshaped recollections.

Myth: You can be spellbound against your will

Spellbinding needs willful patient investment regardless of stories about people being mesmerized without their authorization.

Myth: While you are under a trance, the trance specialist has full power over your conduct.

While individuals frequently feel that their activities under trance appear to happen without their will's impact, a trance specialist can't make you act against your wants.

Myth: You might be super-solid, brisk, or physically gifted with trance.

While mesmerizing can be utilized for execution upgrade, it can't make people more grounded or more athletic than their physical abilities.

Myth: Everyone can be entranced

It is beyond the realm of imagination to expect to entrance everybody. One research shows that it is amazingly hypnotizable around 10 percent of the populace. While it might be attainable to spellbind the rest of the populace, they are more averse to be open to the activity.

Myth: You are responsible for your body during trance

Despite what you see with stage trance, you will remain aware of what you are doing and what you are being mentioned. On the off chance that you would prefer not to do anything under mesmerizing, you're not going to do it.

Myth: Hypnosis is equivalent to rest.

You may look like resting, yet during mesmerizing, you are alert. You're just in a condition of profound unwinding. Your muscles will get limp, your breathing rate will back off, and you may get sleepy.

Myth: When mesmerized, individuals can't lie,

Sleep induction isn't a truth serum in the real world. Even though during subliminal therapy, you are progressively open to a recommendation, regardless, you have through and through freedom and good judgment. Nobody can make you state anything you would prefer not to say — lie or not.

Myth: Many cell phone applications and web recordings empower self-trance, yet they are likely inadequate.

Analysts in a 2013 survey found that such instruments are not ordinarily created by an authorized trance inducer or mesmerizing association. Specialists and subliminal specialists consequently prescribe against utilizing these.

Most likely a myth: entrancing can help you "find" lost recollections

Even though recollections can be recouped during mesmerizing, while in a daze like a state, you might be bound to create false recollections. Along these lines, numerous trance specialists remain distrustful about memory recovery utilizing spellbinding.

The primary concern entrancing holds the stage execution generalizations, alongside clacking chickens and strong artists.

Trance, be that as it may, is a genuine remedial instrument and can be utilized for a few conditions as an elective restorative treatment. This includes the administration of a sleeping disorder, despondency, and agony.

You utilize a trance specialist or subliminal specialist authorized to confide in the technique for guided trance. An organized arrangement will be made to help you accomplish your individual goals.

## Commonly Asked Questions about Hypnosis

Is there a genuine mesmerizing?

Mesmerizing is a genuine strategy for mental treatment. It is now and again misconstrued and not generally utilized. Restorative research, in any case, stays to disclose how and when to utilize trance as an instrument for treatment.

What exactly does hypnosis entail?

Trance is a treatment decision that can help you manage different conditions and treat them. An authorized trance specialist or trance inducer will direct you into a significant unwinding state (now and then portrayed as a daze like a state). They can make recommendations while you are in this state to help you become increasingly open to change or restorative improvement.

Daze like encounters isn't so irregular. On the off chance that you've at any point daydreamed watching a film or wandering off in fantasy land, you've been in a tantamount stupor like condition.

Genuine entrancing or hypnotherapy doesn't require swinging pocket watches, and as a component of a stimulation demonstration, it isn't rehearsed in front of an audience.

Spellbinding is equivalent to hypnotherapy?

Indeed, no, yes. Spellbinding is a remedial treatment instrument that can be utilized. The utilization of this instrument is hypnotherapy. Mesmerizing is to hypnotherapy what canines are for creature treatment, to put it another way.

How Does Hypnosis Work?

A certified trance specialist or subliminal specialist prompts a condition of serious fixation or concentrated consideration during trance. This is a strategy guided by verbal signs and redundancy.

In numerous regards, the stupor like the state you enter may appear to be like rest, yet you are completely aware of what's going on.

Your advisor will make guided proposals to help you achieve your restorative goals while you are in this stupor like state. Since you are in an increased center state, you might be increasingly open to recommendations or proposals that you may incur negligence or get over in your standard mental state.

At the end of the session, your advisor will wake you up from the stupor like state, or you will leave. It's dubious how the impact this extraordinary focus level and thought consideration has. During the daze like state, hypnotherapy may situate the seeds of unmistakable thoughts in your psyche, and rapidly those changes flourish and thrive.

Hypnotherapy can likewise make ready for more profound treatment and acknowledgment. On the off chance that your brain is "jumbled" in your day by day mental express, your psyche will most likely be unable to retain proposals and counsel.

What happens to the brain during a hypnotic session?

Harvard scientists examined 57 individuals' cerebrums during guided trance. They found that: two mind areas in charge of handling and controlling what's going on in your body during mesmerizing show higher movement.

Thus, during entrancing, the locale of your mind that is responsible for your activities and the area that is aware of those activities have all the earmarks of being separated.

Is everything only a misleading impact?

It is possible, yet in the brain's action, trance shows checked differentiations. This shows the mind reacts unmistakably to spellbinding, one that is more grounded than fake treatment.

Like spellbinding, recommendation drives the misleading impact. Guided discourses or any type of social treatment can strongly affect lead and feelings. Entrancing is one of those instruments of treatment.

Do reactions or dangers exist?

Mesmerizing infrequently makes or displays risks to any reactions. It tends to be a safe elective treatment decision as long as the treatment is performed by a certified subliminal specialist or trance inducer.

A few people may encounter gentle to direct symptoms, including cerebral pain tiredness, unsteadiness situational uneasiness. However, an antagonistic practice is

spellbindingly utilized for memory recovery. People who consequently use spellbinding are bound to encounter nervousness, misery, and opposite reactions. You may likewise have a more noteworthy possibility of making false recollections.

Do Doctors prescribe Hypnotism?

A few doctors are not sure that mesmerizing can be utilized for the treatment of emotional well-being or physical torment. Research to advance trance use is getting to be more grounded, yet it isn't being grasped by all doctors.

Numerous medicinal schools don't prepare doctors to utilize entrancing, and during their school years, not all emotional well-being experts get preparing. This leaves plenty of misconceptions among human services specialists about this conceivable treatment.

What is the utilization of mesmerizing?

Trance is advanced for some conditions or issues as a treatment. For a few, however, not all, of the conditions for which it is utilized, inquire about gives some help to utilizing mesmerizing.

Research from confided in sources shows ground-breaking proof that trance can be utilized to treat post-traumatic stress, sleep deprivation, general anxiety disorder or even full-blown depression. Furthermore, trusted sources demonstrate that spellbinding might be utilized to treat:

- Depression and anxiety
- cessation of smoking
- post-employable injury mending
- weight misfortune

More research is required to affirm the impact of trance on the treatment of these and different maladies.

What's in store during a session?

You might not have to spellbind with a subliminal specialist or trance inducer during your first visit. Rather, both of you can discuss your objectives and the procedure they can use to support you.

Your specialist will assist you with relaxing in a happy setting in an entrancing session. They will explain the procedure and audit your session destinations. At that point, dull verbal signs will be utilized to manage you into the stupor like state.

When you are in a daze like the condition of receptivity, your specialist will propose you move in the direction of specific goals, help you envision your future, and guide you towards making more beneficial decisions.

At that point, by taking you back to finish awareness, your specialist will end your daze like state.

Is one session enough?

Albeit one session might be helpful to certain people, with four to five sessions, most specialists will educate you to begin trance treatment. You can talk about after that phase what the number of sessions is required. You can likewise talk about whether you additionally need any support sessions.

# 2. Hypnosis to Choose Health and Quit the Vicious Circle

Welcome to this powerful session to gaining health and becoming the perfect weight and shape, naturally.

Begin your meditation by finding a comfortable place to sit or lie down if you prefer.

Let your arms rest on your knees if you're sitting or by your sides if you are laying down.

Become aware of your fingertips, in particular, your right thumb. Slightly move your right thumb and feel the texture of what your thumb is touching…let your thumb become still.

Bring your focus to your left thumb and move it around a little, noticing what your thumb is touching and how it feels. Then stop…

Now become aware of your right pointer finger…notice the sensation in your fingertip and you move it around ever so slightly. And stop moving this finger.

Bring your awareness to your left pointer finger, moving it around just a little bit…and stop.

Bringing awareness to your right middle finger…notice any sensations here as your slightly move only this finger around…and relax.

Focusing now on your left middle finger, just wiggle only this finger very slightly, noticing the sensations….and relax this finger.

Allow your focus to become centered only on your right ring finger, you can move it just the tiniest amount so that you don't move any other fingers…and stop….

Becoming aware of your left ring finger, moving it ever so slightly…and relax…

Now we have the pinky on the right hand to focus on…move it around a little bit, noting the texture of whatever it lays upon…and stop moving your pinky, bringing your awareness to your left pinky finger…the last one….move it around slightly, noticing how this feels….and stop.

When you stop moving your fingers you notice how relaxed your hands have become.

Your hands guide you through your entire life, choosing things, and lifting things and bringing things home for you. They deserve to relax fully.

Now, if you haven't already allowed, gently close your eyes, and become fully aware of what your hands look like, in your mind.

These hands are so important to your weight loss journey. They are responsible for every food choice that you make. See your hands with your imagination picking up fresh produce from a local farmer's market. This doesn't have to be a real place, you can imagine this farmer's market however you like, but see your hands choosing fresh produce, and fresh herbs. See yourself paying for these items, bringing a smile to the face of the farmer who grew these veggies for you and for everyone.

You have made a wonderful exchange with your hands at this farmer's market. You traded your hard-earned money, for healthy foods that will nourish your body.

Now see yourself arriving at home with these items. You honor the food that you have purchased by cleaning out your fridge from anything that is unhealthy, or old. You can even wipe the shelves in the fridge to cleanse the area for a fresh new start.

See your hands again, making the choices to throw away foods with ingredients that are not good for your body. Your hands hold the items for you to read the labels so that you can make a choice on whether this food is nourishing, or toxic.

See your hands again organizing the freshly grown produce in your fridge, and wherever else you keep your items in your kitchen.

Nice…

You may think it's your mind choosing what you buy. You may think that you have trouble choosing healthy foods, but actually you can just leave it up to your hands to decide what will benefit your overall health.

Now see yourself getting ready to prepare a nutritious meal. Grab some produce or meats from the fridge and feel the coolness that the fridge has brought to these items to keep them fresh for you. Bring some things to your sink that need to be washed, and feel the water washing over these items rinse them, cleaning them for you to eat.

Notice how your hands delicately handle these items because you cherish them. The nutrients that they bring you are literally life-giving. Prepare the veggies by chopping them with your favorite knife, and you can see yourself either cooking them in a pan with a healthy oil or eating them raw.

Just notice how your hands do all this wonderful preparation for you without any effort. You are just enjoying cooking a healthy meal, and your hands complete each task effortlessly.

Your meal is ready to eat, you have cooked yourself a perfectly healthy meal without any junk food or extra bread that you don't actually need. Now see your hands holding a fork and bringing this energizing nutrition to your mouth.

Enjoy this bite that you are imagining right now.

Your hands are amazing at picking out produce that is fresh and juicy. Your hands can feel the texture of things and know when they are perfectly ripe.

Good…

We are going to present you now with a little challenge in this meditation, and you have the choice here to practice something that happens in your daily life.

Imagine that you are being tempted right now with an unhealthy food choice. It could be your favorite dessert at a friend's house, it could be a snack out of a bag at the gas station, or it could be those last items that the grocery stores try to tempt you to buy, right beside the register. Whatever you imagine, you are going to have the choice to see your hands acting in the way you wish them to.

See yourself wanting to reach for this unhealthy food. But instead your hands remain at ease. You can move your fingertips like we did before instead of grabbing the snack. You can see that you didn't need to reach into your wallet or purse to pay for this unhealthy item. Your hands helped you decide what you didn't want to eat.

Great.

Now allow this visual to fade and become aware of your breathing…just notice how you are breathing right now, and inhale just a little bit deeper than you were. Breathe in slowly, and exhale gently.

And when you breathe in say to yourself:

"I choose healthy foods and my hands guide me every time.

My hard-earned money is transformed into healthy foods.

Unhealthy, packaged foods don't end up in my hands, just as my money never pays for these things.

I make choices every day towards a healthy life.

My hands guide me to make a healthy choice, multiple times a day.

Holding healthy food in my hands makes me feel powerful.

Washing and preparing these healthy items makes me feel confident.

My hands help me make delicious healthy food for myself and for others.

I choose health."

Great.

In a moment, take 5 deep breaths, and by doing so you are locking in these wonderful affirmations.

Breathe fully in, see yourself choosing health. And exhale, relaxing your body.

Breathe in as deeply as you can, imagining shopping at healthy places, choosing the freshest items. And exhale, relaxing your body right now as much as you want.

Breathing in seeing your hands again, choosing for you. And exhale, relaxing even more

Inhale deeply, seeing your hands not act upon those unhealthy choices that you used to make. Your hands simply remain still, and do not act upon urges that are unhealthy. And exhale, relaxing very deeply now

Breathing in one last breath, allow whatever comes to mind that benefits your weight loss journey. Be creative. And exhale…only focusing on how relaxed you are right now.

Great. You have done powerful work today.

From now on, your hands are there to guide you, they are no longer under the control of unnecessary urges for unhealthy items. You clearly know when you have an item in your hands, whether you should eat it and absorb the nutrients, or put it back on the shelf, because you know it contributes to weight gain.

# 3. The Role of Hypnosis in Rapid e Permanent Weight Loss

## How hypnosis actually help reduce weight

The most important thing to remember before you learn some basic things about how hypnosis reduces weight is that weight loss is not instantaneous. You will not lose weight in a snap! You will not become sexy and thin after a hypnotist snaps his fingers! But rather it takes a slow, regular process that requires a lot of patience and persistence.

Just like eating the right kind of food or "healthy" food, taking food supplements or even lifting weight, you will never be able to successfully get rid of excess weight in just one sitting. Every aspect of your diet plan, including hypnosis, requires time and a lot of patience to be able to pull through.

But do not despair, it may take a while to gradually lose weight while using diet, exercise and hypnosis but it is a guarantee that you will be able to reap the fruits of your success in no time at all.

## Important things to remember when using hypnosis

Before anything else, here are some important things to do before you indulge in hypnosis

Decide which kind of dieter are you

This is all about figuring out what is actually keeping you from losing weight. Yes, there are millions of reasons why dieters fail but if all these reasons were to be closely considered, all these different reasons would be classified into the following categories:

1. You eat when you want to feel comfort.

Since we were small, our need to take something in our mouth to comfort us has never actually left us. We used to cry when we were hungry and when we needed comfort and our mothers or caregivers where there to immediately answer these needs. As we grew older, we had to mature and take in a lot of different responsibilities but actually, this natural response to anxiety and stress has never left us and we tent do revert to food to seek comfort. This is very much evident when you want to eat your comfort food when you feel depressed or lonely or you tend to eat uncontrollably when you are watching a movie or as you pour your heart out to a friend. If you are an emotional eater, then hypnosis can help.

Hypnosis will help you deal with your emotions and your natural responses to depression and anxiety in a more acceptable manner. You will be able to pinpoint what makes you feel anxious or stressed too and immediately find a more appropriate way to handle it without resorting to overeating or binge eating.

2. Not being true to yourself

We have all gone through believing that we are staying within our diets and exercising the way it should be, but we tend to cheat a little or lie a little just to make us feel a lot better. Why does this happen? There are circumstances every day that affect our daily grind for instance, you overslept and instead of preparing a healthy breakfast, you had no time and just grabbed a latte in a corner coffee shop. You had no time to go to the gym after work that you just grabbed a salad for dinner. You consistently log in a fitness app or keep a close watch of the calories that you eat but you tend to cheat on your diet when you feel depressed thinking it is okay to do so.

All these may not be too much of a fuss and are even trivial matters but when all these excuses and lies add up you will end up not fulfilling your diet goals. You will never be able to fulfill your dreams of getting that slim and sexy body that you have always wanted!

Thus, hypnosis is your key to staying in focus and keeping up with your weight loss plans. When you have learned how to perform hypnosis techniques, you will gain full control over your weight loss plans and reduce being strayed and swayed by different internal and external factors.

3. Thinking food is bad for you

It would be self-explanatory that eating needs to be controlled when a person is on a diet. How else would you be able to control your weight if you continuously eat? However, putting food off and thinking that food is supposed to be bad for you is only going to make it worse. For instance, thinking that fast food is the enemy and you have got to stop eating fast food since it will only make you fat will only make you want it more.

With hypnosis, you will be able to take control of your cravings and not ban food from your life. The key to getting rid of the weight is to learn techniques of how you could develop self- control. You can take a break from your diet plan and reward yourself with a cheeseburger or a regular sundae and this practice allows you to develop self-control and enjoy the food that you love without gaining any weight at all.

4. Do you diet but fail to stick to your exercise plan?

Exercise is an important part of any kind of weight loss plan however there are some factors that could affect the way that we perform this activity. Sometimes we are low on energy, we feel tired and not wanting to sweat it out, we feel very self-conscious when we go out and exercise and sometimes the old manana habit sets in and we convince ourselves that we can start or do it right tomorrow (manana is Spanish for tomorrow). These small mental blocks will eventually build up and will hinder you from starting a healthy exercise regimen.

Hypnosis will help you break down the barriers that are keeping you from exercising and accomplishing your weight loss goals. Hypnosis will help you develop a better and healthier approach to exercise and thus make you one step closer to losing weight.

Do you need a diet or exercise modification?

Now that you would like to use hypnosis for weight loss, it is time to reexamine your weight loss strategies. Here are a few things to help you determine if your diet plan and exercise plan is indeed the best one for you:

1. Is your diet and exercise plan according to your particular health condition? Do you suffer from medical conditions such as high blood pressure, diabetes, arthritis or thyroid conditions? If you are following a weight loss plan that is according to your medical needs, then good for you. Hypnosis will make you more focused on your goals which will eventually help you lose weight and even conquer your medical condition.

2. Do you feel tired and out of energy after following your diet and exercise regimen? If you feel this way after a week or more of indulging in your weight loss plan, then you should re-evaluate your strategies and have a professional look into your diet plan and exercise regimen. Dieting does not have to leave you tired, weak and tingling and exercise should never leave you sore, out of breath and weak afterwards! After consulting with a professional and setting all things right about your diet and exercises, you will be able to use hypnosis to bring you closer to your goals.

3. Do you tend to put off exercise more than often? If you tend to cheat and just forget about exercise, then you should think about getting a professional to train you. The only way that you can

focus on your exercise regimen is that you should first understand why you are doing routines and how these could benefit you. By training under the guidance of a professional and by using hypnotherapy you will be able to get hold of yourself and start training seriously. You will be able to exercise with conviction when you have your mind, your body and your spirit ready to commit!

There may be more questions running through your mind and so if you have a pen and paper handy, list these down. Sit and rethink, is your diet plan working for you? Would you rather use another diet? Would you rather exercise at home or in a gym? Consider your answers before starting on hypnosis for weight loss.

Look for a professional hypnotist

Needless to say, that you need to find a professional that will help you with conquering your weight loss goals. Finding a professional to help you could be a challenge since there are many out there that offer outrageous claims. So how do you find a legit and experienced hypnotist?

1. Check on the hypnotist's profile online or search for references online. Never rely on someone claiming to "reduce weight fast" or "gain control overeating in just seconds." Remember that weight loss and eating right takes time and hypnosis is simply used to guide dieters and to help dieters gain control over their emotions towards eating and exercising.

2. Look for candidates from your doctor or family physician. A hospital–recommended hypnotist is not just reliable but is experienced in dealing with different kinds of medical conditions and thus could help you out successfully. Check for the hypnotist's years of experience and ask if he has handled weight loss cases before.

3. Look for candidates from family and friends. A recommended professional is welcome, but you should still double check on his experience and if he has handled cases just like yours.

4. Look for potential candidates from hypnotherapist associations in your area. In the US, there is the American Hypnosis Association which offers learning materials, certification and help for anyone interested in learning hypnosis. The association is the largest national association of hypnotherapist as well as professionals that practice hypnosis. You will be able to find recommended hypnotists that work in your area and even offer distance learning, residency programs and free classes on the subject.

# 4. Gastric Band with Hypnosis

There are many different types of hypnosis that benefits the human body in different ways. Some of these methods include hypnosis for weight loss and healthy living, which are different types of hypnosis for weight loss. Gastric band hypnotherapy is one of them and popularly known as a type of hypnotic state that is suggested to your subconscious, which involves fitting a gastric band around your stomach. This in return helps you lose weight, along with general hypnosis for weight loss sessions.

This type of hypnotherapy is often considered as the final type of hypnotherapy people try if they would like to reach their goals. The practice involves surgery known as gastric band surgery. During surgery, a gastric band gets fitted around the upper part of your stomach, with the purpose to limit the total amount of food you consume daily. This is a more extreme type of hypnotherapy for weight loss, which has proven to help people lose weight. Since it is surgical, you cannot carry out this method yourself. It also includes potential risks, which is why it must be treated with respect and only carried out by a certified medical practitioner.

You can, however, implement gastric band hypnotherapy yourself. It is a technique most commonly used by hypnotherapists with the purpose to trick the subconscious in believing that a gastric band has been fitted when in reality it hasn't. Since hypnotherapy is focused on putting your conscious mind on silent, and implementing thoughts and beliefs in your subconscious mind, as a type of hypnotherapy, it is quite effective. Given that hypnotherapy offers us many benefits, as well as allow us to imagine and come to terms with what we are capable of doing, it acts as the perfect solution to reaching some of your goals that may seem out of reach.

Gastric band hypnotherapy involves the process of believing that you have experienced the physical surgery itself, ultimately making you believe that the size of your stomach itself has been reduced too.

The gastric band used in gastric band fitting surgery is an adjustable silicone structure, used as a device to lose weight. This gastric band is used during surgery and placed strategically around the top part of your stomach, leaving a small space above the device. The space left open above the gastric band restricts the total amount of food that is stored inside the stomach. This is done to implement proper portion control every day and prevents overeating. The fitted gastric band physically makes it difficult for one to consume large amounts of food, which can set you in the habit of implementing proper portion control daily. This will essentially cause you to feel fuller after eating less, which in return encourages weight loss.

Most people choose to have the surgery after they've tried other methods to lose weight, including yo-yo dieting, diet supplements or over the counter drugs, all with the hope to lose weight. Gastric band surgery acts as a final resort for those who desperately want to lose weight and have been struggling for a long time.

Gastric band hypnotherapy serves as a very useful method as it can allow you to obtain a similar result as the gastric band fitting surgery itself. That's because you are literally visualizing getting the same procedure done and how you benefit from it. During gastric band hypnosis, you are visualizing yourself losing weight subconsciously, which translates into your conscious reality.

Hypnotherapists that specialize in gastric band hypnotherapy focus on finding the root of what prevents their clients from losing weight. Most of the time, they discover that emotional eating is one of the leading causes that contribute to people holding on to their weight. They also make a point of addressing experiences that remains in your subconscious mind but is yet to be addressed. These experiences often cause people to turn toward unmindful and emotional eating, which then develops into a pattern that feels impossible to kick.

Since stress is added to our lives every day, and people don't stop and take the time to process feelings or perhaps not even give it a thought, most turn to food for comfort. This also plays into emotional eating, which has extremely negative effects on the body long-term as it also contributes as one of the leading causes of obesity.

Given that obesity is an incredibly bad illness and more people get diagnosed with the condition every day, it is something that needs to be addressed. If gastric band hypnotherapy can prevent it or restructure our thinking patterns to not act on our emotions, but rather invite and process it, then it is a solution that everyone who needs to lose weight should try.

Once a hypnotherapist learns about why you're struggling to implement proper portion control, they will address it with the virtual gastric band treatment at a subconscious level. During this visualization session, you will have imagined that you have undergone the operation and had the gastric band placed around your upper stomach. This will lead you to think that you feel fuller quicker, serving as a safer option opposed to the surgery.

## How gastric band hypnotherapy works

Hypnotherapy for weight loss, particularly for portion control, is great because it allows you to focus on creating a healthier version of yourself safely.

When gastric band fitted surgery gets recommended to people, usually because diets, weight loss supplements, and workout routines don't seem to work for them, they may become skeptical about getting the surgery done.

Nobody wants to undergo unnecessary surgery, and you shouldn't have to either. Just because you struggle to stick to a diet, workout routine or lack motivation, does not mean that an extreme procedure like surgery, is the only option. In fact, thinking that it is the only option you have left, is crazy.

Some hypnotherapists suggest that diets don't work at all. Well, if you're motivated and find it easy to stick to a diet plan and workout routine, then you should be fine. However, if you're suffering from obesity or overweight and don't have the necessary drive and motivation needed, then you're likely to fail. When people find the courage and determination to recognize that they need to lose weight or actually push themselves to do it, but continuously fail, that's when they tend to give up.

Gastric band hypnotherapy uses relaxation techniques, which is designed to alter your way of thinking about the weight you need to lose, provides you a foundation to stand on and reach your goals, and also constantly reminds you of why you're indeed doing what you're doing. It is necessary to develop your way of thinking past where you're at in this current moment and evolve far beyond your expectations.

Diets are also more focused on temporary lifestyle changes rather than permanent and sustainable ones, which is why it isn't considered realistic at all. Unless you change your mind, you will always remain in a rut that involves first losing, and then possibly gaining weight back repeatedly. Some may even throw in the towel completely.

Since your mind is incredibly powerful, it will allow you to accept any ideas or suggestions made during your hypnosis gastric band hypnosis session. This can result in changing your behavior permanently as the ideas practiced during the session will translate into the reality of your conscious mind. By educating yourself on healthy habits, proper nutrition and exercise, you also stand a better chance of reaching your weight loss goals sustainably.

The gastric band fitting procedure will require a consultation with your hypnotherapist where you will discuss what it is you would like to gain from hypnotherapy. After establishing your current health status, positive and negative habits, lifestyle, daily struggles, and goals, they will recommend the duration of hypnotherapy you will require to see results. During this time, you need to inform your hypnotherapist of your diet and physical activity history. They are likely to ask you questions about your current lifestyle and whether you changed it over the years. If you've lived a healthy lifestyle before, then they will try to find and address the reasons why you let go of yourself and your health. If you have always lived your current unhealthy and unbalanced lifestyle, they will trace it back through the years with the hope to discover the reasons behind it. During your initial session, your weight loss attempts, eating habits, and any health issues you may experience will be addressed. Your attitude toward food will also be acknowledged, as well as your relationship with it, with people, and your surroundings.

Now your therapist will have a better idea of the type of treatment you need. The procedure is designed to have you experience the gastric band surgery subconsciously, as though it has really taken place. You will be talked to in a deep, relaxed state, exactly the same as standard hypnosis. During this session, you will be aware of everything happening around you. Suggestions to help boost your self-esteem and confidence are often also incorporated into the session, which can also assist you in what you would like to achieve consciously.

You will be taken through the procedure step-by-step. Your hypnotherapist may also make theater noises to convince your subconscious even more. After your session, your hypnotherapist may give you self-hypnosis guides and techniques to help you practice a similar session for the results to become more effective. Sometimes, gastric band hypnotherapy only requires a few sessions, depending on what your needs are.

Gastric band hypnosis doesn't only involve having to go to physical hypnotherapy sessions, but it also requires you to implement some type of weight management program that specifically addresses your nutrition, addiction, and exercise habits. It addresses habits between your body and mind and helps you implement new constructive ones.

After gastric band hypnosis, you can expect to feel as though you have a much healthier relationship with food, as well as a more mindful approach in everything you do. During the visualization process of gastric band fitting surgery, you will come to believe that your stomach has shrunk, which will trick your brain to think that you need less food. This will also make you think that you don't need a lot of food, which will make you more acquainted with consuming healthier portion sizes.

Gastric band hypnotherapy is successful as it makes you think that you are full after eating the daily recommended amount of food for your body. It is also considered much healthier than overeating or binge eating. You will learn to recognize the sensation of hunger versus being full, which will help you articulate between the two and cultivate healthier eating habits.

## Types of gastric banding techniques used in hypnotherapy for weight loss

- Sleeve gastrectomy - This procedure involves physically removing half of a patient's stomach to leave behind space, which is usually the size of a banana. When this part of the stomach is taken out, it cannot be reversed. This may seem like one of the most extreme types of gastric band surgeries, and due to its level of extremity, it also presents a lot of risks. When the reasons why the sleeve gastrectomy is done and gets reviewed, it may not seem worth it. However, it has become one of the most popular methods used in surgery, as a restrictive means of reducing a patient's appetite. It is particularly helpful to those who suffer from obesity. It has a high success rate with very few complications, according to medical practitioners. Those who have had the surgery have experienced losing up to 50% of their total weight, which is quite a lot for someone suffering from obesity. It is equally helpful to those who suffer from compulsive eating disorders, like binge eating. When you have the procedure done, your surgeon will make either a very large or a few small incisions in the abdomen. The physical recovery of this procedure may take up to six weeks. (WebMD, n.d.)

- Vertical banded gastroplasty - This gastric band procedure, also known as VBG, involves the same band used during the sleeve gastrectomy, which is placed around the stomach. The stomach is then stapled above the band to form a small pouch, which in some sense shrinks the stomach to produce the same effects. The procedure has been noted as a successful one to lose weight compared to many other types of weight-loss surgeries. Even though compared to the sleeve gastrectomy, it may seem like a less complicated surgery, it has a higher complication rate. That is why it is considered far less common. Until today, there are only 5% of bariatric surgeons perform this particular gastric band surgery. Nevertheless, it is known for producing results and can still be used in hypnotherapy to produce similar results without the complications.

- Mixed Surgery (Restrictive and Malabsorptive) - This type of gastric band surgery forms a crucial part of most types of weight loss surgeries. It is more commonly referred to as gastric bypass and is done first, prior to other weight-loss surgeries. It also involves stapling the stomach and creates a shape of an intestine down the line of your stomach. This is done to ensure the patient consumes less food, referred to as restrictive mixed surgery, combined with malabsorptive surgery, meaning to absorb less food in the body.

## What you need to know about hypnotic gastric band therapy

If you're wondering whether gastric band surgery is right for you, you may want to consider getting the hypnotherapy version thereof. Hypnotherapy is the perfect alternative, is 100% safe as opposed to surgery which has many complications, and also a lot more affordable. It has a success rate of more than 90% in patients, which is why more people prefer it over gastric band surgery. Given that you can also conduct it in the comfort of your own home, you don't even have to worry about the cost involved. Overall, it serves as a very convenient way to slim down, essentially shrinking your stomach.

Again, hypnosis doesn't involve any physical procedure involving surgery. It is a safe alternative that uses innovative and developed technology to help you get where you want to be. The hypnotherapy session involves visualizing a virtual gastric band being fitted around your stomach that allows you to have the same experience as you initially would during surgery, but without the discomfort, excessive costs and inconvenience.

The effect is feeling as if you are hungry for longer periods, require less food, and experiencing a feeling of being full, even if you've only eaten half of your regular-sized portion. This will also help you make healthier choices and discover that you can indeed develop a much healthier relationship with food then you currently have.

If you're wondering whether gastric band hypnotherapy will work for you, you have to ask yourself whether you have the imagination to support your session. Now, of course, everybody has an imagination, but is yours reasonable enough?

If you can close your eyes and imagine yourself looking at something in front of you that is not there, and spend time focusing on it, then you can make it through gastric band hypnotherapy successfully.

It's normal to think before you start anything, that if it isn't tailored to you specifically, it is likely to fail. However, visual gastric band hypnosis can offer you emotional healing. This supports your goals, including weight loss and health restoration. If you spend time engaging in it, you will learn that you can achieve whatever you set your intention on. You can remove your cravings subconsciously, eliminate any negative and emotional stress, as well as memories that form a part of your emotional eating pattern. Given that emotionality forms a big part of weight gain, you should know that it can be removed from your conscious mind through hypnotherapy and serve any individual willing to try it.

Gastric band hypnotherapy has a 95% success rate among patients, according to a clinical study conducted in the U.K. This study also proved that most people will be able to accept and succeed in hypnotherapy, but if they're not open to the experience, they won't find it helpful at all. People who are too closed off from new ideas, like hypnotherapy, which is often made out to be a negative practice among the uneducated, won't be able to relax properly for a hypnotherapist's words to take effect. (Engle, 2019)

After just one hypnotherapy session, you will know if it works, as it is supposed to start working after just one session. That is why hypnotherapy is not recommended for everyone. It's only suggested to anyone ready to change their feelings toward food. If you don't believe in it or that it will get you to where you want to go on your weight loss journey, it is deemed useless.

The cost of gastric band hypnotherapy sessions with a professional hypnotherapist can only be established after you've undergone an evaluation. Usually, every new patient requires up to five sessions in person. During these sessions, energy therapy techniques are also taught, which will help assist any struggle a patient may have with anxiety, anger, stress, and any other negative emotion.

# 5. Evidence that Hypnosis is Useful

The best way to describe the experience of hypnosis is to view it as a type of therapy that focuses on controlled attention. It's not something that feels scary or out of the ordinary. Those who are apprehensive should consider giving it a shot at least once before debunking the practice altogether. It's something that can benefit you by allowing you to change your habits healthily.

Is there a negative side to hypnosis? It depends on how you perceive the practice, as well as additional features it encompasses.

For some, it may be a wonderful experience, but for others, not. Since it's not an invasive procedure, and you're not taking something physically to lose weight, it may come across as a fad. If you're the type of person who struggles to stick to something or can't see beyond what's in front of you, then chances are it may not be your cup of tea.

Also, unless you have the willpower to engage in self-hypnosis consistently, you will have to visit a hypnotherapist to receive hypnotherapy sessions. Professional sessions can cost anywhere between $100 to $250 an hour. Considering that you have to engage in hypnosis for at least three months to see proper results, it's easy to see why people may quit at the get-go. Since most insurance companies refrain from covering hypnosis, it will also have to come out of your pocket.

On a positive note, if you can't afford professional hypnotherapy sessions, you can find countless guides, articles, and podcasts like this one online. If you can manage to put in the necessary time required to succeed in losing weight or simply kick some of your bad habits, then you will be thrilled to find that it is indeed very effective. Although three months of practice seems incredibly long, you will reach your goals in no time. Plus, you'll do it in a sustainable self-sufficient manner, which is also a bonus for your self-development.

Often, when people can't lose weight, it is because they are unmotivated and deprived of a positive and disciplined mindset.

Hypnosis manages to target specific factors that cause weight gain. In a sustainable manner, hypnosis helps you overcome those negative influencing factors, which can present itself as quite challenging to face daily.

Challenges may include anxiety disorders, depression, stress, fear, negative eating habits, such as overeating or consuming a low-calorie diet and addictive habits, such as smoking and consuming alcohol.

Hypnosis is a passive-aggressive approach to solving problems people face in their daily lives, but generally they don't know how to deal with them. It alters our minds to change the way we respond and react and can aid as a healthy tool to guide us through our daily struggles, worries, and just about any situation with ease. Since unmindful eating, such as overeating or even a bulimic disorder, are usually influenced by emotional reactions, it's becoming clear why hypnosis could work for those who suffer from any type of related disorder. Adding self-image into the mix, it's equally understandable why a person's self-image can be rectified with hypnotherapy. Once the individual's mind is altered to accept themselves, care for themselves and treat their bodies as something valuable, only then will they be inclined to take better care of themselves. This goes hand-in-hand with what they consume every day and the effort they are more likely to put in to feel good and not only look good.

Focusing on the right things, such as health rather than image, can shift your mindset significantly. It's like focusing on making money in your career instead of obtaining overall happiness in your life. If you're not happy, then making money will just be a temporary escape or solution to your problems. However, if you spend time doing what you love and are really passionate about it, instead of doing something you potentially don't like because you're making money from it, the long-term results will be quite negative. Since we only get one body, one machine to operate with, we as humans must be inclined to look after it.

People are also more likely to find it difficult to maintain a healthy lifestyle if they have low self-esteem.

This contributes to the reason why hypnosis is so effective and considering that you can do it all by yourself instead of seeing a hypnotherapist, gives you no excuse to not engage in some manner of self-healing through hypnotherapy. It can be just as effective carried out by yourself as it is presented by a professional.

By adopting a healthier mind to consume better food and improve your lifestyle, also comes the responsibility to learn more about healthy living. Even if you're in the healthy mindset of wanting to eat a balanced diet, what do you actually know about doing it? Sure, every day we are presented with countless advertising campaigns and food products that pushes the following terms:

- Low fat
- No sugar
- 25+ added vitamins
- Low caloric deficit

However, are these disclaimers really what we should be looking for on the packaging labels of our food?

Not whatsoever. The last thing you should be eating is artificially induced foods, with package labels that suggest that vitamins or minerals has been added to it. The same goes for the label "no sugar." We don't know whether you've given it a thought, but why does that yogurt taste so sweet?

Is it magic? Well, of course not, but it has definitely been pumped with something that's not good for you. Some of the most common artificial sweeteners include aspartame and xylitol, which can have serious negative effects on your long-term health if consumed daily. Yet food brands don't disclaim that on their labels, do they?

When undergoing hypnotherapy with the purpose of becoming healthier or to lose weight, you can't just visit your hypnotherapist or conduct the session yourself. You have to implement a process that will support new intentions, such as eating healthier. There are countless eBooks, podcasts, and cookbooks available online and in-store to help you to maintain a sustainable diet. If you're really uncertain about what to do, it's always a good idea to ask your medical practitioner. Having your blood tested for certain allergies or intolerances, such as dairy, glucose, and wheat can also be quite helpful in guiding you with what you should and shouldn't eat.

The best way to lose weight, of course, is to maintain a consistent balance of 80% nutrition and 20% physical activity. To lose weight effectively and permanently with hypnosis, you have to follow the 80:20 rule ratio.

Hypnosis works for weight loss, but only if you devote yourself and maintain a healthy balanced lifestyle. Again, it's important to remember that hypnosis is not a diet or quick solution that will get you to where you want to be. Instead, it's a tool that can be used to support your weight loss journey by rectifying old habits and possibly creating new sustainable ones.

Providing you with raw evidence of someone losing weight as a result of hypnosis by displaying a before and after photo isn't a very reasonable tactic, either.

Anyone can post pictures online and promote a weight loss method. However, trying it out, you'll start to notice a more mindful version of yourself, which won't only translate in your relationship on how to approach food, exercise or your lifestyle, but it will also show in the way you treat and take care of yourself.

At the end of the day, our bodies serve as vessels that carry us through life. How well we look after it, is entirely up to us.

# 6. Portion Control Hypnosis

Overcoming binge eating is not something that will happen in one day. Binge eating is a disorder and an illness. We say this not to discourage you, but to make certain that you do not underestimate the problem. That said, it is most certainly worth it to try to deal with this problem, for not only does it limit opportunities, when you no longer suffer from it, but you'll also find your life improved in many ways.

- Weight loss – better than all those diets you've been trying, controlling your binge eating will significantly cut down the calories and lead to weight loss. Of course, it will, after all, you'll no longer be filling yourself up on junk food (which quite often seems to be the go-to foodstuff of the binge eater).

- Higher self-worth – When you control your urges instead of your urges controlling you, you'll find that you feel better and that the shame, guilt and low self-esteem issues you've been dealing with will lessen significantly if not disappear entirely.

- Social engagement – Once you're feeling better about yourself and you don't feel the need to lock yourself away to eat for several hours, you'll find more opportunities for social engagement. And this will lead to far greater mental and physical health being. We are, after all, a social species.

- Greater life satisfaction – Bad is stronger than good. With that, we mean that negative things occupy far more of our attention. Also, a bad habit far outweighs something equally good within minds. Thus, overcoming something negative like binge eating can tremendously improve your life satisfaction. This goes double when you consider how proud you'll be of overcoming such a large problem.

## The Dangers of Over-Eating

On the other hand, if you continue to binge eat the consequences can be catastrophic as you get locked into a self-destructive spiral where your binge eating provokes greater self-loathing and that in turn provokes greater binge eating. Binge eating is quite often a coping mechanism for the problem's life keeps hurtling our way. The problem is that it doesn't just help you cope, but it also provokes new problems like social isolation, obesity and a negative self-image, which in turn require you to work harder to cope.

And that's not even mentioning the actual mental and health problems that this disorder can cause, such as:

- Low self-esteem issues and feeling bad about your life or yourself
- Low quality of life
- Depression
- Anxiety
- Feelings of social isolation
- Bipolar disorder
- Substance abuse
- Problems managing your workload, as well as functioning in your personal life or in social situations
- Obesity and the medical conditions associated with therewith, such as:
- type 2 diabetes

- joint problems
- heart disease
- gastroesophageal reflux disease (GERD)
- sleep-related breathing disorders like sleep apnea

## Why Do I Binge Eat?

There are a lot of contributing factors to binge eating. Binge eaters, for example, are often quite perfectionistic and very hard on themselves. They often have trouble accepting any weakness in their character and focus on the negative rather than the positive. They also have a tendency to see things in black and white terms. This means that there is no 'almost succeeded' in their vocabulary. There is only success and failure. We all fail occasionally, but the binge eater takes this especially badly.

Often, they also have an obsession with dieting, calorie counting and losing weight. This can frequently lead to them forbidding certain foods for themselves, including but not limited to all the foods they actually enjoy eating. Then when they do indulge, as they're not certain when is the next time they'll be able to eat these foods, they can keep going, trying to fill up to fulfill that forbidden food urge for the period to come.

Putting that aside for the moment, you'll find that there are normally triggers for binge eating and similar problems. Binge eating is often a coping mechanism. For that reason, there are often things that make it happen. These triggers might cause anxiety, stress or other factors which affect self-worth.

## Proven Strategies to Overcome Binge Eating

For this reason, consider keeping a binge-eating diary. You don't need much for this; a standard planner will do (depending on how often you binge eat, really). In it track what caused you to binge eat. You'll be surprised with how quickly you'll start noticing patterns that you might otherwise have been completely unaware of. Often just a week is enough. Armed with this knowledge you'll then have a much better picture of what it is that is setting you off.

## Manage Stress

As you'll notice from your diary, your cues are often stressed, or anxiety related. The first thing you, therefore, need to do is eliminate as many of these stress factors. Your work is setting off binge eating? Don't take your work home with you. Talk with the in-house psychologist about what stress management suggestions they might have.

And if all that doesn't work, consider finding a new job. Perhaps it's a social situation with a loved one? If you believe they're open for a conversation about such topics suggest, without accusation, that you find interacting with them stressful and that this is affecting you negatively. If you don't think they're capable of this kind of a conversation without judging you or causing you to discomfort, then perhaps consider taking some time away.

Where you can't eliminate stress, manage it instead. There are stress-management strategies that can help. These include meditation, exercise as well as fun and relaxation. These are all healthy ways to reduce the effects of stress in your life and if you can manage to replace your binge eating with any or all of these activities that might already help.

## Plan on Eating Three Meals a Day

Don't skip breakfast. This is something that quite a lot of binge eaters do, and it plays right into their binge eating. It has been shown that people that do not eat breakfast are more at risk of heart attacks and are more likely to be overweight than those who do eat breakfast. So, all those health benefits you were thinking you were getting, they aren't there.

How does avoiding breakfast do all these things? The reason is twofold. First off, by skipping breakfast you're continuing the fast from the preceding evening onwards. Or, put more succinctly, you're starving yourself for longer. This causes all kinds of stress responses in your body, which aren't healthy and actually lead to calorie retention as your body slows down calorie consumption in order to help you cope. Then, when you do eat, because of your hunger it's going to be far harder to resist junk food cravings and eat healthily. Finally, it can lead to a disconnect between your stomach and your mind.

So, the long and the short of it is, eat breakfast! Try to take in at least some fruit and perhaps a bowl of cereal in the morning. From there try to expand your breakfast into something healthy that will keep you satisfied until lunch.

Also don't skip lunch or dinner. Plan to get three square meals a day that give you the nutrition and the satisfaction that you need. That last part is important. If you're not enjoying the food you're eating, then there's a good chance you'll use that as an unconscious excuse to indulge (read binge eat) at some point along the line. This is not to say that you should eat burgers every day, but it does mean that you don't have to eat your boring vegetable salad every day either. Make certain that there are certain aspects of what you're eating that you enjoy.

### Enjoy healthy snacks

It's also a good idea to have healthy snacks on hand for when you have a craving for something. Again, this does not mean 'boring'. You're not trying to punish yourself. That will ultimately just trigger another episode of binge eating. Instead, look for something you like. There are quite a few snacks available on the market nowadays that are actually quite tasty without being loaded up with sugar, salt or fat. This includes fruit but might also include nutritional bars and nuts. It depends on what you like really.

## Establish stable, healthy eating patterns

Stability is your friend. For that reason, try to make arrangements so that you eat at regular times, preferably with other people as mealtimes are great occasions to socialize. If you don't have anybody to eat with, don't worry. That will change once you're back to a more normal and healthy ritual.

The first step towards that goal is to standardize your mealtimes so that your body once again gets used to more normal rhythms. This will allow your brain and your stomach to reconnect and thereby make you more aware of when you are hungry and when you're satiated. This will make it easier to stop when you need to. Also, don't eat in front of the TV. When you do so, you're more likely to overeat as it takes longer for you to become of signals from your stomach telling you that you've had enough.

## Avoid Temptation

Your life will be a lot easier if you can avoid temptation. There are several ways to do this. The most obvious one is to not have junk food in the house. This does not mean you can never have junk food. Indulging occasionally is fine. In this case, however, only buy enough of the product that you're craving, not enough that you can hide some away (chances are you won't anyway).

If you live with somebody else who occasionally like to have junk food in the house, talk with them and ask them to help you overcome your problem. Yes, that does mean asking them not to keep junk food lying around where you can find it. It doesn't have to be permanent, just until you've got your binge eating under control.

In order to avoid temptation when you're in the supermarket or in other places, don't go shopping when you're hungry. This is a very valuable piece of advice that won't just help your binge eating problems but will also help you avoid overspending, as everything always seems far more enticing when we haven't eaten. So, before you go to the supermarket or the mall, make sure you have a meal. This will make the entire experience far easier for you personally and for your wallet as well.

## Stop Dieting

Yes, you read that right. Don't diet. Chances are it's making your binge eating worse and it doesn't really help that much anyway. So, cut it out. Instead, start trying to eat in a way that's healthier in the long run. This means you focus on getting enough fruit, vegetables, protein, fiber, and vitamins.

The great thing about eating in this way is that it's more positive. When you focus on getting the right foodstuff, you're not focusing on what you shouldn't eat, but rather on what you should. The human mind isn't very good at 'no'. This is easily demonstrated with the following experiment. Don't think of a white polar bear. What happened when I said that? Chances are you immediately thought of white polar bear.

The same thing happens when you try to exclude certain foods from your diet. The very act of excluding them makes you focus on them. And that, in turn, means that you've got to use precious will power to not indulge.

This will only work for so long until the dam breaks, at which point it's very hard to stop yourself from thinking – subconsciously or consciously – oh what the hell, let's go all the way. So, don't diet.

## Exercise

There is very little in this world that exercise isn't good for. It fights negative attitudes; helps you lose weight and generally makes you feel better about your situation by flooding your system with endorphins and other happy chemicals. What's more, it will help you fight both boredom and stress, get to bed on time and improve your energy levels. And though you might not believe it in the beginning when you're just getting started and your body is not used to it, many people find it quite enjoyable!

The trick is to exercise and not torture yourself. A lot of people, including trainers, seem to believe that the only way to gain is through the pain. That is nonsense. The only thing that will cause is for you to hate exercising and feel resentful. That won't benefit anybody.

Instead, a much better strategy is to start off slowly and then build up. In this way, you won't feel resentful for what you're doing, and you'll have the enjoyment of seeing an improving line. Sure, this does mean that it will take a little longer before the effects of the exercise start to show, but on the flip side, it also means that the chance you'll keep going is much more significant.

If you weren't doing any kind of exercise, start by going walking or riding a bike. Initially, it doesn't have to be that far, as long as you've got a steady rate of improvement built in. Today a mile, tomorrow a mile and a quarter. After that, think about joining in with a group. Here again, it's important that you don't go overboard and join the super hardcore do or die group, but something more at your level. Water aerobics, stretching exercises or other forms that will push you but not break you are the best to start out with.

If you are obese or overweight, initially you might not see much weight loss. Don't worry about that. You're still changing. It's just happening on the inside. You'll be transforming fat to muscle, for example. Only after that, the actual weight loss will start setting in. Don't get discouraged. Instead, look at what you can do, rather than how slim you are. Perhaps keep an exercise calendar in which you track what you did and how you feel. Then, consider you're at least straining yourself; you should see steady improvement.

Dealing with Boredom and Avoiding 'No'

It isn't just in terms of food that you should avoid the 'no' word, you should avoid it as a whole. So, don't just exclude binge eating from your life, find an alternative way to fill your time. So, take up a hobby. Better yet, continue a hobby that you used to have but had to let go as a result of binge eating – something you really enjoyed, and you feel you should be able to enjoy again. In other words, fill your time. Otherwise, boredom will set in and then you'll spend your time trying (and failing) to not think about binge eating.

Get other people involved. Join a team or a class where other people come to depend, you're your presence. This way, even if you're having a down day, you'll be far more likely to go. Before you go you might not believe that you can actually enjoy yourself, but that will often change once you get there. In psychology, we call this the hot-cold empathy gap. It means that we can't imagine how something will feel unless we're feeling it. Its why temptation is so hard to resist and why we can't believe we can't resist it when we're not feeling it.

It's also why we can't imagine enjoying something outside of the house if we're sitting in it depressed and unhappy, but once we're outside of the house we find it quite easy to enjoy ourselves. And it is the reason why it's a good idea to take up activities where it isn't just our expectation of enjoyment that will get us to go, but also social commitments.

You could also consider getting a dog. These can offer you a great deal of companionship and also offer you opportunities to go for walks, which is obviously a great way to get exercise. Now, this goes without saying, but you must actually want a dog, as they do require a lot of attention and love. Don't get one if you're not sure about it, as otherwise, you'll feel bad about yourself and about not taking care of the dog!

If you are considering getting a dog, may I advise astray rather than a thoroughbred? Your local pound will have dogs that need homes or will be put down otherwise. Save yourself by saving a dog. It has a nice ring to it, doesn't it?

Alternatively, reach out to friends and family. It doesn't matter if you've lost touch. That is, in fact, probably a better reason to reach out to them.

Don't just send them an email or a chat message either. Actually, take the time to talk to them over the phone or in person. Now the goal here is not to tell them all about your problems, but rather just enjoy spending time in the company of others. This is an incredibly effective technique for feeling better and without a doubt one of the easiest ways to feel better about ourselves. Give it a try!

# 7. Hypnosis Weight Loss Session

Welcome to the weight loss hypnosis session, which can be conducted in the comfort of your home or just about anywhere you won't be likely to experience interruptions. Given that hypnosis requires you to be completely focused on your thoughts, preferably in silence, you will need to find a space where this is attainable.

Getting rid of potentially interrupting objects, such as your smartphone or any digital device and noise is necessary for you to take in the complete experience. Without focus, you will not be able to access a quiet space in your mind and will be constantly distracted.

Apart from physical surroundings and creating a tranquil or quiet environment, it's also best to ensure you practice hypnosis for weight loss without people around or any noise. It's also best to choose a space where you feel safe and content before you start your practice. Returning to this space every day around the same time will help you to develop the habit of practicing hypnosis daily and stick to a routine. Without consistency, hypnosis won't produce the necessary results required to aid in your weight loss journey. All these factors are important to take note of before starting your hypnosis for weight-loss session.

Since you're reading this, you are obviously interested in what hypnosis for weight loss has to offer you, and given that you've chosen weight loss as a specified solution to help you in your daily life, good for you to decide to implement change.

Although kickstarting a journey like this, whether it's 21-days or up to three months, may seem difficult to follow through until the end, I hope this session will inspire you to keep coming back for more.

This session includes a 21-day guided meditation plan, which is specifically designed to help you develop a habit. After these three weeks, you are more likely to want to engage in some form of hypnotherapy daily as it will have proven to serve you positively.

That's the thing with doing something really beneficial for you, much like hypnosis, often, you are hesitant to do it unless you've managed to develop a routine. This routine must, of course, be sustainable and in some sense either enjoyable or feel like it's positively affecting your day. The same goes for exercising, your daily eating habits, and any methods you may implement to rid your body and mind of stress.

Now, although 21-days of benefiting your physical health and mental well-being doesn't necessarily present itself as a challenge, most individuals can't commit to any practice that lasts as long as three weeks. However, if you take a moment to consider the benefits you will reap after three weeks, even entering the habitual period thereafter, it may become easier to adopt hypnosis as a part of your daily routine toward healthy living.

Given that hypnosis is focused on creating new habits and replacing bad ones, you'll find that it can be quite addictive once you've managed to quiet your mind. We, as humans, most definitely require some time to wind down and destress after busy days spent in the midst of stress, which persists all throughout our lives. In today's fast-paced world, it's very uncommon to not experience some form of stress, anxiety, or even depression in our lives. Stress specifically, is one of the biggest contributing factors why people gain weight.

Hypnosis is often compared to meditating. Looking at the similarities, it's easy to see why this makes sense. Since people often struggle to meditate, with the main issue being struggling to calm their minds, hypnosis may present itself as a difficult challenge to start.

However, with persistence, this will surely get better. Something is changing your attitude and the way you perceive different factors in your life, including the difficulty of quieting your mind, which can spark significant change in your reality.

This, of course, is not "The Secret," yet it has countless similarities and characteristics that present the same outcome for those who try it. If you think about what causes you to develop bad habits, you will find that it is primarily stress or teachings instilled in you from a young age. If you think about what causes you to overeat, as an example, you will easily believe that hypnosis can indeed lead you to turn that habit around.

Since we tend to rush through our daily lives, including work and our duties at home, we don't slow down to take the time to look after ourselves.

There are a lot of different components integrated into how we think, feel, and what we prioritize. Usually, we don't prioritize ourselves, which is why people tend to "let go of themselves." Considering that it's also much easier to quit or choose the easy route, rather than spending time looking after ourselves, preparing meals or getting active and moving our bodies as it was designed to do, it's clear that shifting your mind is the answer. Even though losing weight or changing your daily routine, waking up early, feeding your body the right foods, etc., seems like a lot of obstacles placed in your way, it's really just all in your mind.

That is why the best practice you could ever engage in starts with overcoming barriers in your mind, and, ultimately, taking control of it. It's not rocket science, and when you're in it, you'll discover that if you affirm a new idea of what you'd like to be or have in your life, you will obtain it.

## How to use hypnosis to change eating habits

1. Think yourself thin and implement affirmations to help you get there in a healthy and sustainable way by adopting the habits of people who have already reached their weight and body positivity goals.

2. Adjust your mind to assist your weight loss goals and support it every day.

3. Don't eat without thinking, which includes both emotional eating, binge eating, or any act of mindless eating. Recognize the differences between emotional eating and eating because you are hungry.

4. Enjoy cooking and fill your home with good food instead of anything tempting. This will also help you to develop more controlled eating patterns. By not filling your home with sugary or fatty foods, you're instantly making a change. Although it's difficult, it's a bold one to be proud of.

5. Don't eat because of comfort; that usually leads to the over-consumption of calories.

6. Don't be reckless. If you're going to spend most of your time sitting in front of a television binge-watching your favorite series, you're bound to want to snack. Stay true to your affirmations and believes during hypnosis and remind yourself to stay active throughout the day. This will prevent eating out of boredom and potentially lead to more weight-loss.

7. Stay motivated throughout your journey with hypnosis. Remembering that you're not going to achieve results overnight, but in the long haul, it is the answer to keeping both your mind and body in check.

## How to conduct hypnosis the right way

Self-hypnotization can do wonders for your health and may also sound far too good to be true. However, many experts believe that changing our thought processes can lead to a much better state of health and quality of life.

To prepare yourself for this practice, you should:

## Focus on now instead of thinking about tomorrow

The future will always exist, but it's not something we can control, is it? Sure, we can control most things that influence it and builds up to it, but we cannot control much else. Often, the things we want and hope for, or even work for, don't always reflect back to us along the line or according to our planned timeline. Given that we are not in control of what lies ahead, there's no need to be worried about it. Giving the wrong things too much energy without knowing where it's going will instill the idea into our minds that we are not in control of our life. On that note, unless you're in control, can you really thrive? Can you really focus on the present? In essence, can you be happy or reach your goals? Thinking in this sense also translates in the context of today. Should you start on Monday–a day that is idealized as the perfect day to start something challenging or should you just start today, the day you can control?

## Jump into reality

The average human is extremely fixated on overthinking, and this is something that we don't necessarily feel like we have any control over. However, thinking about overcoming the habit of thinking too much may not even feel reasonable to some. Given that people who overthink are also considered much more emotional than others, hypnosis for weight loss can help individuals to overcome more than just bad habits related to their diet and lifestyle. It can also help them overcome the habit of overthinking a workout, planning too much, as well as obsessing over their calorie intake. With hypnosis, you will be able to rid your mind of overthinking processes and make healthier choices, which can get you a lot farther than thinking about everything you want, or still need to do. Finally, focusing on how your body feels when it's moving or even how it feels when it's consuming the right nutrients will trick your mind in wanting to implement change that will beneficially serve your body.

## Detox your emotional state of mind

Anyone who is overweight, suffering from obesity or other eating disorders, is bound to have some type of emotional issue. Call it an emotional barrier, but it is something that holds most people back from losing weight. People don't struggle with weight loss because they are necessarily unaware of what to do. In fact, they may even know exactly what it is they must do but convince themselves that they can't get themselves to do it because of underlying emotional issues, which also translates into excuses and bad habits. Professional therapists will often prescribe their clients to feel their feelings instead of just supresing it. Once you feel and embrace it, you can finally make use of it and let it go. This will, in return, set your body up for success as you will be able to focus on what's good for you instead of holding on to what's not.

## Implement powerful breathing techniques

Integrating powerful breathing, including diaphragmatic breathing is wonderful for amplifying your focus. When we focus on deep or controlled breathing, both our minds and bodies enter a state of being calm, allowing us to feel like we are in control. This also opens the door to feeling happier, allowing us to implement more positive habits and experiences into our days, rather than just going through a motion rut. Focusing on diaphragmatic breathing causes you to breathe deeply, which when you breath out, tightens and flattens your stomach. This not only relaxes your body but also creates the idea of visualization that you can indeed have a flat stomach. Apart from diaphragmatic breathing, you should also try out Buteyko breathing. This type of breathing involves breathing small quantities of fresh air in and out of your nose, which reduces the total amount of oxygen you use. Given that most individuals over-breathe, they can't control their bodies when they are stressed. This contributes to bad digestion, inadequate sleeping patterns, and many other negative habits that contribute to weight gain. Implementing this breathing technique can solve one issue you struggle with but can translate into solving countless other issues you face. It will also reduce anxiety and place you in a more mindful state of living.

# 8. Hypnosis for Weight Loss Mini Habits

We all have habits that we partake in that aren't always in the best interest of our overall health. Some of them you might realize, others you might not always recognize just how ingrained into your life they are. If you really want to live a life centered around losing weight, then it's important that you are focused on better habits.

Habits start small. You won't always change overnight, but miniscule progress will always be better than none at all. It's time to recognize bad habits and turn them into good ones so that you will be able to fulfill your biggest weight loss fantasies.

## Mini Habits Hypnosis

If you want to climb a set of stairs, you are going to do so one step at a time. You have to start introducing mini habits in order for you to lose weight. You are going to enter a hypnotic state. You are going to stay focused and relaxed in order to feel these messages deeper, on a more important level. You are going to remain calm and centered on the things that are most important in your life. Your mind is clear, and you are ready for all the things that are going to come your way in this journey.

You are becoming more and more relaxed, more and more centered. You are thinking only of yourself, your body, your mind, your soul. You are only thinking about these things in this present moment. You are not thinking about work, school, family, friends, or anything else in your life. You are only thinking about you.

You are focused more on yourself by paying attention to your breathing. You are centered on who you are, feeling the air come into your body and leave slowly. You are feeling your lungs fill with air and you feel the way that it leaves your body as well. You are feeling light, airy, and free. You are becoming more and more relaxed.

You are going to start to make good decisions for your health. You aren't going to make any choices that hurt you. You aren't going to make any decisions that will hinder your health. You are going to stay completely centered on making the best choices for your body.

You are going to have a plan every day. You are going to know what needs to be done that will help you contribute to your weight loss goal that day. You will have an idea of the food that needs to be eaten. You are going to have a regimen for what you need to do to work out.

You are feeling more and more relaxed knowing now that you have a plan. You are feeling at peace with the goals that you have because you know the steps that it will take to achieve them. You feel a calmness and serenity as you become more and more focused on getting the things that you want in this life.

You aren't going to make any decisions based on your emotions. You are going to fight through even the most challenging of feelings. When you are presented with the feeling of wanting to indulge in a snack, you are going to make sure that you choose a healthier option. You are going to choose to eat smaller portions.

You are going to have strong willpower and you will know how to say no.

You are going to do all of this because it is good for your health. You are still feeling yourself breathing, in and out, in and out. You are feeling the air come into your body, and you feel as it leaves as well.

You are only thinking about your health. You are only concerned with the healthiest options. You are only focused on the things you need to do to bring you peace and serenity with your body.

You are going to say no to impulses. You understand now that the urge to eat another snack or to skip the gym is based on emotion. These are based on impulses. You are not going to make decisions based on these feelings anymore. You are only going to make choices centered around your health. You are going to always decide to do what the best thing for your body is.

You are going to resist your biggest urges. You are going to instead put your focus on helping yourself push through the emotional reactions. You are going to go to the gym even when you feel like staying home. You are going to skip that snack even when you have the biggest craving.

You feel your air continue to be regulated. Breathing like this reminds you that you have the power over your body. You are going to remember the importance of breathing like this throughout your weight loss journey. You are aware of the power that you have to change the way that you physically feel. This power starts with your breath.

You feel as it comes in through your nose, and as it leaves through your mouth. You understand that this breathing will help you work through your impulses. This breathing will help you stay focused at the gym.

All of this is going to help you achieve your goals. The choices that you make are most important for fulfilling your fantasies. Everything that you do for your body is a choice. Every time you eat, move your body, sleep, and feel stress, there will be a choice.

You will not always have the ability to control what choices you have. You will always have an option. There will always be an option that is best for your health.

You are going to always look for the option that is going to make you feel best overall. You are going to look past momentary desires. You are going to push through urges to give in. You will not fall victim to your impulses anymore. You are going to stay centered and focused on your health.

You are feeling the air come into your body and leave. You are feeling the way that the air spreads throughout the rest of your body. You are aware of how this makes all of your limbs feel. You can feel the air come into every aspect that makes you the person that you are now. You feel full. You feel complete. You feel like yourself, you feel strong.

You are going to make better choices. You are going to include healthy habits. You are going to always look for ways to grow your health. You are revolving around your body. You are listening to impulses. You are choosing to confront your inner challenges in the healthiest way possible.

You feel the air enter and exit your body. As you count down from twenty in your mind, you are going to solidify all of the ideas that you have when it comes to controlling your body and your impulses.

Ten, nine, eight, seven, six, five, four, three, two, one.

# 9. Self Hypnosis Session

## How to Do Self-Hypnosis

There are several ways that you can do self-hypnosis. In fact, there are three main ways that will work for this kind of problem. Before we get into the advantages and disadvantages of each method, let's first discuss using an actual live hypnotherapist to lead you through your session. Although self-hypnosis is the least expensive route, as well as being the one that many people choose because of self-consciousness, there is some value in having an actual person hypnotize you, especially a qualified hypnotherapist who has dealt with these kind of problems in the past.

Benefits of Using a Hypnotherapist

There are a number of benefits to using an actual hypnotherapist instead of doing self-hypnosis. There are some pretty compelling reasons to get an actual therapist to do the session if you can afford it, and you find someone you can trust.

First of all, a hypnotherapist is different from a hypnotist. Hypnotherapists may be actual psychologists or have some other kind of education. Even if that isn't the case, hypnotherapists that operate a hypnosis clinic full-time will have a great deal more experience dealing with issues than those who do not.

Hypnotherapists usually have solid plans for treating disorders like overeating. They may specialize in one specific type of hypnosis or they may be able to do a variety of hypnotic sessions. Generally, they are safe, trustworthy and able to help.

However, the real benefit of using a hypnotherapist is that you can customize your sessions to target the beliefs or thoughts that you want to change. It might be difficult to do this with self-hypnosis, and hypnotherapists have a higher success rate when they can work one on one with a client and create a customized hypnosis session for whatever behavior they want to modify.

Self-Hypnosis

If you decide to do self-hypnosis instead, you can still gain enormous benefits. The first method of self-hypnosis is a guided session with yourself. Put yourself into a light trance state where you will be able to communicate clearer suggestions to yourself about the beliefs, thoughts and actions that you want to change.

1. Start by sitting comfortably as with any hypnosis session and loosening or removing any restrictive clothing.

2. Second, start taking deep breaths and tell yourself to become relaxed. Try to imagine a peaceful serene place and put yourself there. This might be a spot out in the woods, a place on a beach with the waves lapping gently at your feet, or it might simply be an empty room with white walls.

3. Once you are relaxed and feel as if you are starting to float, or you feel somewhat detached from yourself, begin giving yourself the suggestions that you have written out in advance. Continue this until you are awake and alert again, or until you have fallen so deeply into trance that you can no longer make the suggestions.

4. A couple of tips: Many people ask if this method is dangerous – if the hypnotic session that you are inducing will continue indefinitely if no one is there to bring you out of it. The answer is no. The most that will happen is you will fall asleep eventually. Also, if you are having a hard time relaxing, you might try some meditation music to help you get into a state of suggestibility.

## Customized Self-Hypnosis Sessions

The second method of doing hypnosis is to have someone create a customized hypnosis session. This will generally require you to provide or edit a script to add your own suggestions that you want to focus on.

Once you have a customized script, you will need to find someone to record it. Some people like to ask a friend to record it, and if you have someone who has a clear speaking voice and a decent microphone this is fine. However, if your friend recording the session is not confident, or mispronounces words or has other pauses, halts or noises in the session it will not be effective.

Your other option is to have a professional hypnotist or voice artist record your session. This will obviously cost money, but it is a much more effective way to create your self-hypnosis sessions. One tip that may save you a little money is to find a website that offers pre-recorded hypnosis sessions and get them to put your suggestions into some of their sessions. The induction can remain the same, but the suggestions for overeating can be your own script. This will be much fewer words and will cost a lot less.

It is probably not going to work if you record the hypnosis session yourself. No matter how high quality the session is, getting into a trance state using your own voice is very difficult, because it is one that you hear in your head all the time. It is much more effective to have someone else record it for you.

## Pre-recorded Hypnosis Sessions

The final option for self-hypnosis is finding hypnosis sessions online that fit your particular problem. There are many websites that offer free sessions, and there are even a large number of sessions on YouTube and other sites. The session doesn't have to have your custom script in it to be effective. Obviously, using your own suggestions will be much more keenly targeted than a generic one, but if you have no other option this treatment will still have the potential to make some great changes in your behavior.

## Self-Hypnosis Session

Start by taking a deep breath in…. then let it out slowly. Make sure that you are seated comfortably and that you are somewhere safe where you can relax for twenty minutes or so. During this session you will ignore all daily noises like the telephone ringing, traffic sounds outside or any other sounds except for sounds of alarm. If you hear an alarming sound you will immediately come out of the trance state with no residual sleepiness.

Relax…. take another breath in….and out. Let go of all of the stress that you are holding onto. Relax…. breathe in….and out.

Start by relaxing the muscles in your feet and legs. Think of each muscle one by one and let them all just let go and relax. Feel a warmth spreading from your toes up your calves…. feel the warmth go to your thighs and as it moves across your body feel each muscle group that it reaches completely let go and relax.

Relax your stomach muscles….and moving up to your chest and shoulders. feel the warmth move up your body and relax…. breathe in…and out…now your neck muscles are feeling warm and relaxed. Feel all of the muscles in your face relax completely.

Imagine yourself at the top of an escalator. As you step onto the escalator, you realize that you are passing numbers on white signs on the way down. The first number is 10. As you pass each number you will fall deeper and deeper into a relaxed state. Take another deep breath in….9…..the escalator is moving you slowly forward and down…8…..you are becoming more and more relaxed each time you pass a number…7…..relax your body completely and let go of everything….6….you reach the halfway point of the slow moving escalator…5…you are very relaxed now…completely relaxed…4…..you feel as if you are floating down the escalator becoming more and more relaxed…3….you can see the bottom and when you reach it you will become even more deeply relaxed than you are now..2…..you reach the bottom of the escalator…1……breathe in…and out….very relaxed now….

With each of the suggestions that I give to you, you will become more deeply relaxed than before. Each of these suggestions will stay in your subconscious and they will be used to influence your behavior when you awake…. continue to relax as each suggestion is given….

You no longer have to eat too much food to feel the good feelings about yourself that the food provides…. your feelings are good as they are…

When you feel an emotion, your response is to eat. However, you don't need to do that. When you feel anxiety, you should slow down and try to find the cause. You don't need to overeat to solve anxiety. Overeating will not solve the problem; it will only make it worse. If you feel depressed, that means that it is time to spring into action. When you feel frustrated, what you have been doing may not be working and instead of eating, try something else. If you feel stressed, you will not become less stressed by eating. Instead, try to relax and take things one by one as they come. If you feel the emotion of loneliness, try to surround yourself with people instead of food.

Eating will not satisfy these emotions. When you feel these emotions, your response will be to do something other than eating. In the future, you will find it easier to understand these emotions and you will not feel compelled to eat. Your feelings are there to guide you through life and each one means something different. Your response to these will no longer be to eat. Instead, you will allow each emotion to happen and then take action.

In the future, you will be free from the cycle that you have fallen into in the past. Eating will not solve any problems, even temporarily, and will only make you feel worse. Eating should only be done when you are hungry, and you should eat until you are no longer hungry. When you find yourself tempted to make large portions, you will have the willpower to say no and you will be very satisfied with the amount you have.

When you have other emotions, they are not hunger. Those are simply emotions and eating will not make them go away. You will remember these things when you awake. As I count up from 1 you will start to feel more awake, but still remembering all the suggestions given…2….you are coming up…3…..you are starting to feel less relaxed and more alert…4….when you awake at the end of the count, you will feel refreshed and ready to continue your daily activities…5…you are more awake now…6….7….8….9….you will wake up completely refreshed on the number 10…..

# 10.Deep Sleep Hypnosis Sessions

Although you might be tired, you may still struggle to actually fall asleep because you aren't able to become fully relaxed. Going to bed doesn't mean just jumping under the covers and closing your eyes. You will also want to ensure that you are keeping up with incorporating relaxation techniques into your bedtime routine so you can stay better focused on getting a complete rest, not one that is constantly disturbed by anxious thoughts.

The following meditation is good for anyone who is about to go to bed. You will want to include this for getting a night of deep sleep, or one that will last for several hours. Keep your eyes closed, and ensure the lighting is right so that there is nothing that will distract you from falling asleep. No lighting is best, but if you do prefer to have some sort of light on, ensure that it is soft yellow or purple/pink. Always choose small lights and nightlights instead of overhead lighting.

## Better Sleep Guided Hypnosis

You are in a completely relaxed place, ready to start the process of falling asleep. You are able to stretch your body out, feeling no strain in any limb, muscle, or joint. You are not holding onto any stress within your body. Your eyes are closed, and there is nothing that you need to be worried about in this present moment. You have given yourself permission to fall asleep. You are allowing yourself to take time to relax. You have granted your soul the ability to become completely at ease before falling asleep.

Become aware of your breathing now. Feel how the air moves in and out of you without any effort on your part. Every move that you make is one that helps you to bring in clean, healthy air. In everything that you do throughout the day, your lungs are always working hard to push you through. Everything that requires more strain means making your lungs work harder. Now, we are going to give them a bit of rest, as well. They can never fully stop, but we are going to give them the long, deep, clean, and relaxing breaths that they need now.

Counting while you breathe will help you to become even more relaxed. Breathe in for one, two, three, four, and five. Breathe out for six, seven, eight, nine, and ten.

Once more, this time breathing in through your nose and out through your mouth. Breathe in for ten, nine, eight, seven, six, and out for five, four, three, two, and one.

You are feeling refreshed. You are focused. You are centered. You are at peace.

As thoughts pass into your head, allow them to simply float away. When you think of something that does not pertain to this moment, simply push the thought away. Imagine that you are in a pool and a bug is on the surface of the water. What would you do? At the very least, you would push it away. Gently push your thoughts in another direction and allow them to float away.

Think of your thoughts as if they were sheep jumping over a fence. Imagine them escaping from the pasture in which they are held, only to jump away and go somewhere unknown. Watch as your thoughts hop over the fence. They are passing from your mind out into the world. You are simply releasing them, doing nothing more.

Your thoughts are the stars burning brightly above. They are scary, they are beautiful, and they will always eventually burn out. You will never rid yourself of your thoughts. They will always be dotting the sky. They are so distant, however. They are slow burning. Do not reach for the stars, simply let them be. Let your thoughts slowly burn out now. You only need to be focused on relaxing and becoming more and more at peace.

Feel how you are becoming more and more relaxed. You are letting go of tension in every part of your body. You are becoming more and more focused on centering yourself. You are becoming closer and closer to sleep. You are getting this rest to prepare for the day tomorrow. What happens tomorrow will happen then. There is nothing that you can do about it now. Worrying and stressing isn't going to help you whatsoever. What will help you the most at this moment is drifting deeply into a heavy sleep. Give your body the rest that it needs.

The earth is all asleep now as well. Don't just feel how you are becoming more relaxed. Feel the way that the earth has been tucked into bed as well. Feel how it is now dark and how others are sleeping restfully just as you are. There are some just waking, and some still awake, but they will eventually rest just as you are now. It is time for you to become a part of this whole peaceful earth.

Nothing about the future is scary. You have survived thus far. You are not worried about what is going to happen tomorrow, or the day after, or the day after. Even the bad things that might happen will eventually fade just as well. Nothing is going to keep you from sleeping at this moment. No amount of anxiety will keep you awake.

Everything tomorrow will be unknown. You can prepare but never predict. You are prepared. The best way to ensure that it will be a good day is to get some rest. Allow yourself to get this sleep. Give yourself permission to enjoy this deep and heavy sleep as it exists at this moment.

You are completely comfortable, all throughout your body. You feel relaxation everywhere and you exude peace and serenity.

You are feeling more and more relaxed from the top of your head to the bottom of your toes. You feel your mind start to fade into a dreamlike state. You are feeling as though there is nothing that will keep you awake.

Feel your jawline relax. You hold onto so much tension that you don't even realize. Not now. Not at this moment. You are releasing yourself from all physical strain.

Allow your ears and forehead to be as still and as relaxed as possible. These are heavy and can hold a ton of tension. At this moment, you are letting them become as relaxed as possible. Nothing is going to keep the muscles in your head so tense.

Be aware of the way that we hold our muscles throughout the rest of our bodies. Allow yourself to become relaxed. And even further. And even further. Even when we try to relax, we don't let go of our bodies all of the way. Give yourself to rest. Devote yourself to sleep. Marry the idea of being peaceful.

Allow every bone to become still, relaxed, and serene. You are tranquil from the inside out. You are rested from the outside in.

Let your shoulders relax as much as possible. Feel how they become heavy on your pillow. Your shoulders can hold the weight of the world. It can feel like everything in your body is pressing onto them. Let these shoulders drop deeper and deeper, further and further.

Let your hips be relaxed as well. Your waist, your abdomen—all of this will also hold tension. Release those feelings. Let your body become calm and still. Allow yourself to be relaxed all over your entire body.

Feel the calm spread from your mind down all the way to your toes. The peace is like butter, you are the warm toast. Spread it throughout and allow it to melt into you. Let your body fade away, slowly becoming more and more peaceful.

Feel your stomach rise as you are breathing. You are breathing slower and slower, keeping your heart rate low as well. This will make it easier to fall into a deep and healthy sleep.

You are becoming more and more relaxed. You are starting to feel your body become completely calm. Not one single part of you is still holding onto any tension.

Nothing about the past or the future scares you.

It is time now to fall asleep.

You are going to get the deepest sleep by letting everything go. You are not carrying any fear, anxiety, stress, or pain. You are at peace. You are content. You are calm. You are complete. You are tranquil.

Don't allow thoughts to keep you at the surface of your sleep. Become more and more tired, getting closer and closer to falling all the way asleep.

We are going to count down from ten. When we reach one, you will be fast asleep.

Ten, nine, eight, seven, six, five, four, three, two, one.

## Meditation for Deeper and Healthier Sleep

One of the best ways to really become relaxed and find the peace needed for better sleep is through the use of a visualization technique. For this, you will want to ensure that you are in a completely relaxing and comfortable place. This reading will help you be more centered on the moment, alleviate anxiety, and wind down before bed.

Listen to it as you are falling asleep, whether it's at night or if you are simply taking a nap. Ensure the lighting is right and remove all other distractions that will keep you from becoming completely relaxed.

Meditation for a Full Night's Sleep

You are laying in a completely comfortable position right now. Your body is well rested, and you are prepared to drift deeply into sleep. The deeper you sleep, the healthier you feel when you wake up.

Your eyes are closed, and the only thing that you are responsible for now is falling asleep. There isn't anything you should be worried about other than becoming well-rested. You are going to be able to do this through this guided meditation into another world.

It will be the transition between your waking life and a place where you are going to fall into a deep and heavy sleep. You are becoming more and more relaxed, ready to fall into a trance-like state where you can drift into a healthy sleep.

Start by counting down slowly. Use your breathing in fives in order to help you become more and more asleep.

Breathe in for ten, nine, eight, seven, six, and out for five, four, three, two, and one. Repeat this once more. Breathe in for ten, nine, eight, seven, six, and out for five, four, three, two, and one.

You are now more and more relaxed, more and more prepared for a night of deep and heavy sleep. You are drifting away, faster and faster, deeper and deeper, closer and closer to a heavy sleep. You see nothing as you let your mind wander.

You are not fantasizing about anything. You are not worried about what has happened today, or even farther back in your past. You are not afraid of what might be there going forward. You are not fearful of anything in the future that is causing you panic.

You are highly aware within this moment that everything will be OK. Nothing matters but your breathing and your relaxation. Everything in front of you is peaceful. You are filled with serenity and you exude calmness. You only think about what is happening in the present moment where you are becoming more and more at peace.

Your mind is blank. You see nothing but black. You are fading faster and faster, deeper and deeper, further and further. You are getting close to being completely relaxed, but right now, you are OK with sitting here peacefully.

You aren't rushing to sleep because you need to wind down before bed. You don't want to go to bed with anxious thoughts and have nightmares all night about the things that you are fearing. The only thing that you are concerning yourself with at this moment is getting nice and relaxed before it's time to start to sleep.

You see nothing in front of you other than a small white light. That light becomes a bit bigger and bigger. As it grows, you start to see that you are inside a vehicle. You are laying on your bed, everything around you are still there. Only, when you look up, you see that there is a large open window, with several computers and wheels out in front of you.

You realize that you are in a spaceship floating peacefully through the sky. It is on autopilot, and there is nothing that you have to worry about as you are floating up in this spaceship. You look out above you and see that the night sky is more gorgeous than you ever could have imagined.

All that surrounds you is nothing but beauty. There are bright stars twinkling against a black backdrop. You can make out some of the planets. They are all different than you would ever have imagined. Some are bright purple, others are blue. There are detailed swirls and stripes that you didn't know were there.

You relax and feel yourself floating up in this space. When you are here, everything seems so small. You still have problems back home on Earth, but they are so distant that they are almost not real. There are issues that make you feel as though the world is ending, but you see now that the entire universe is still doing fine, no matter what might be happening in your life. You are not concerned with any issues right now.

You are soaking up all that is around you. You are so far separated from Earth, and it's crazy to think about just how much space is out there for you to explore. You are relaxed, looking around. There are shooting stars all in the distance. There are floating rocks passing by your ship. You are floating around, feeling dreamier and dreamier.

You are passing over Earth again, getting close to going back home. You are going to be sent right back into your room, falling more heavily with each breath you take back into sleep. You are getting closer and closer to drifting away.

You pass over the earth and look down to see all of the beauty that exists. The green and blue swirl together, white clouds above that make such an interesting pattern. Everything below looks like a painting. It does not look real.

You get closer and closer, floating so delicately in your small spaceship. The ride is not bumpy. It is not bothering you.

You are floating over the city now. You see random lights flicker on. It doesn't look like a map anymore like when you are so high above.

You are looking down and seeing that gentle lights still flash here and there, but for the most part, the city is winding down. Everyone is drifting faster and faster to sleep. You are getting closer and closer to your home.

You see that everything is peaceful below you. The sun will rise again, and tomorrow will start. For now, the only thing that you can do is prepare and rest for what might be to come.

You are more and more relaxed now, drifting further and further into sleep.

You are still focused on your breathing; it is becoming slower and slower. You are close to drifting away to sleep now.

When we reach one, you will drift off deep into sleep.

Ten, nine, eight, seven, six, five, four, three, two, one.

# 11. Binge Eating Problem: Who Binges?

A difference between the person who suffers from binge eating disorder (BED) and the person who has issues with other eating disorders is that there is no self-induced vomiting. The person who binges doesn't show signs of so-called "compensatory behavior", which means that they don't go exercising too much after they eat nor do they decide to vomit immediately after the meal to avoid gaining weight. Therefore, it is not surprising that most of those who binge also have issues with obesity or are overweight.

So, who binges?

Those who eat frequently without any control. As we already explained, those who suffer from binge eating disorder eat enormous amounts of food and without proper breaks between meals. When having a binge-eating episode, a person is unable to stop eating even if they want to do so. Their need for uncontrolled eating is stronger than their will to stop at that moment.

Those who binge have certain eating habits that can be identified. The simplest ones are quick eating or eating large amounts of food without being actually (physically) hungry. This also includes the necessity to eat even if they start feeling uncomfortable because they have already passed the point of being full.

People who binge often feel shame and guilt. These emotions are typical of those with binge eating problems. These feelings are frequently caused by the amount and way of eating they have during their binge episodes that we already mentioned above. Binging is used to confront challenging emotional states, and it is usually caused by stress or boredom and anger.

Binging also means that a person will have certain behavior around food. As we just explained, those who suffer from binge eating disorder use it to deal with different emotions, and because of that, they can develop eating habits that are a bit different. For example, many of those who have BED prefer eating alone, and they don't feel comfortable with having others around while they are eating.

However, this doesn't mean that everyone who eats too much or doesn't like to eat in front of others suffers from binge eating disorder. There are certain criteria that one must meet to be diagnosed with this eating disorder. Some of the clearest symptoms are:

There has to be a certain period in which a person eats excessive amounts of food. These periods in which one eats large portions of food are known as binge episodes (we mentioned them as one of the key characteristics of those who binge). This criterion includes loss of control over their eating and the fact that they can't stop the episode.

Now, eating a lot in a short amount of time can happen even without having BED. That is why we would like to point out a few more characteristics that a person should have to be diagnosed with binge eating problem:

- The binge episode eating will normally be much faster than normal eating.
- A person can even feel uncomfortable because he or she has already eaten too much, but that doesn't stop them.
- There is no physical hunger when the person starts having a binge episode
- Binge eaters suffer embarrassment about the way they eat and the amount eaten during a binge episode, which is why people with BED prefer to eat alone.

- They experience feelings of guilt, disgust, and depression. People who suffer from binge eating disorder often have a bad attitude about themselves after their binge episodes.

There is a certain pattern that has to be followed to be sure that a person is potentially suffering from BED. It is usual that they have a binge episode at least once each week for a period in excess of three months. Otherwise, it can be seen as stress eating without health consequences that can be too serious.

Another serious eating disorder that has spread through the world is called bulimia nervosa. However, there is one major difference between bulimia nervosa and BED. Unlike the first disorder, the binge-eating problem doesn't involve extreme behaviors that are related to weight loss. As we mentioned, professionally, these behaviors are known as "compensatory", and they are often extreme and can end up having permanent and serious consequences. Still, if a person suffers from a disorder known as anorexia nervosa, it is not uncommon for the following symptoms, which include binge eating ones. And while it is true that anorexia nervosa involves extreme dieting it doesn't mean that it automatically excludes binge-eating problems as a diagnosis either.

The most recent statistics say that approximately 3.5% of females have binge eating problems in the USA. When it comes to men and adolescents, about 2% of men and 1.6% of adolescents have issues with this eating disorder. BED can be developed regardless of the ethnicity or race of the person. Still, we can point out a few groups that can be more vulnerable to binge eating disorder than others.

Firstly, people who are dieting frequently have bigger chances of ending up binge eating. Some researchers say that the chances are even 12 times bigger than for those who don't use any dieting programs. Also, it is scientifically proven that BED has a bigger impact on younger people rather than on older people. The average age for developing BED is between the early and mid-twenties. However, that doesn't mean that older people (especially women) don't have binge eating problems.

Two out of three people dealing with binge eating issues are obese. Nevertheless, being overweight is not the only health risk that comes from BED. Obesity, in general, can be a cause for many health problems like increased levels of cholesterol or high blood pressure. Furthermore, there are several types of cancer that obese people can suffer from such cancers as kidney cancer, pancreatic cancer, breast cancer, uterine cancer, thyroid cancer, and so forth. For females, obesity can cause problems with the menstrual cycle. Long-term, this means that being overweight can prevent their ovulation, which can make it hard for women to have children.

# 12. Why You Should Not Binge-Eat

If you are a binge-eater, then you acknowledge that you must have known that there was a need for you to stop the habit before picking up this. At the very least, you have shown understanding that you realize that your binge episodes need to stop. Getting rid of binge-eating is not that straightforward, though. As a real psychological disorder, it goes beyond just the realms of nutrition, deficiencies, and physical discomfort. It also brings attendant social problems, health problem, and possibly personality disorders.

Let us take a look at some of the ill-effects of binge-eating.

Weight gain

This is perhaps the main reason why most people with BED seek to get rid of it. Binge-eating confers on you a first-class ticket to excessive weight gain in very short order. It is an express route to pile on extra pounds of flesh that you would be better off not gaining.

A conservative estimate puts the figure of people that are on weight loss programs due to BED at forty percent. That means for every ten individual that starts a weight loss program; four could have stopped themselves the stress by discarding binge-eating a long time ago. Even more incriminatingly than, as high as twenty percent of all obese people can trace their weight problems to bingeing.

A study by Walden Behavioral Care Center theorizes that the average amount of calories consumed by binge-eaters per episode is 3,415. In addition, twenty percent of people with BED will consume 5,000 calories in a typical episode. Ten percent will consume approximately 6,000 calories in a single episode. These figures serve to illustrate just how badly binge-eating skews the amount of food (in calories) that you may consume in a day. Of course, the excess food will do only one thing; blow your weight out of proportion.

With the excessive increase in weight comes a whole list of weight issues. If for any reason, excessive weight gain is a primary candidate for why you should not make binge-eating a recurrent habit for you.

Even with people who do not gain weight despite binge-eating, there is a danger. It is typical for such people to believe that since they are not overweight, there is no need to seek treatment. This leaves the disorder to exacerbate. Therefore, regardless of your weight range, BED still poses a danger to your general wellbeing.

Loss of self-esteem

As with many of its effects and causes, it is hard to appropriately determine if it is low self-esteem that causes binge eating, or a loss of esteem is only a symptom of binge-eating. However, what is very sure is that binge-eating and a loss of self-respect always walk together hand-in-hand. In a perpetual vicious cycle, a binge-eater is likely to feel angry and stupid for overeating. These negative emotions give rise to a usually vitriolic self-tirade that does nothing to improve self-worth. Bingeing leaves you feeling helpless and unworthy of a healthy lifestyle. It leaves you feeling inferior for not being able to exert any control over what you put in your mind. Especially when the ill effects such as weight gain and health problems start to arise, you are almost unable to forgive yourself. Sadly, not even the reduced esteem can force one off the wagon. In most cases, it deepens it.

Eat, feel disgusted with yourself, promise to change, eat in excess again, feel even more troubled, and then turn to food to feel better. It continues like that with each episode further shaving off some of the self-esteem you should be enjoying. The only way to end the disgust, and destroy the inferiority complex is to get rid of binge-eating.

Social awkwardness

This is a by-product of low self-esteem brought about by overeating. Having a negative image of yourself often spills over to the way you handle yourself in public and social encounters. Our external body language is built to mirror the internal feelings we have. Therefore, if binge-eating is taking a hammer to your mental health and confidence, it is bound to show up negatively in the way you interact with others. This exacerbates further when such encounters occur around the time you just binged. Bingeing often happens under an air of secrecy too, and the levels of uneasiness from your eating sessions can spill over to the first few social encounters you get after it.

Lower levels of productivity

An imbalanced mental state automatically translates to lower levels of productivity at work. Add to that the fact that physical discomfort that follows binges can render you unfit for work for some time and BED provides economic impact too. The Health Economics undertook a research to compare productivity levels in obese people and individuals that fall within a normal weight range. The results were instructing. The income of obese people was down 2.5% when compared to people with normal body weight. In any case, keeping up binge-eating is surely going to rack up some extra bills on food and consumables with time.

Digestion problems

Our body is built to specification. It has limits to what it can take and process at once. Food undergoes a sophisticated process that leads to its digestion and eventual absorption for use. However, BED disturbs this system. By eating so much food within a short period of time, you get to overwhelm this system and cause it to function at less than optimal conditions. Acid reflux, for instance, is more common with binge-eaters. The excess food too can rob you of efficient digestion and cause constipation. At the same time, rapid gastric emptying where the body gets rid of most of the food you have consumed without processing it for nutrients is likelier with binge-eating. I am trying to tell you that binge-eating does your digestion process no favors.

Physical discomfort

There is no point over-flogging this issue. We all know just how comfortable our stomachs can feel when we overeat. Pain, rumbling, and distension of the abdomen are not the most favorable outcomes that should accompany eating, but excessive food comes with that.

Health issues

If you are not trying to stop binge-eating because of weight, then the chances are high that you are trying to stop BED because of the inherent health risks it comes along with. Think obesity and the health complications it comes with, then give same to binge-eating disorder. Consider low self-esteem and the wrong health-affecting lifestyle choices it can provide and ascribe the same to binge eating. Binge eating affects your health in some of the ways below;

-Cardiovascular problems

Think the heart and the cardiovascular system. Then, think excessive damage to them if you keep up binge-eating. Cardiovascular diseases and conditions such as heart attacks, hypertension, and stroke are the leading causes of death worldwide, and diet contributes a lot to their development. Binge-eating causes an overall increase in the level of triglycerides, cholesterol, and total body fat content, all indices that raise the chance of developing a sudden heart attack. Forget the technical language; all I am saying is the more you binge-eat, the higher your chances of having cardiovascular challenges.

-Diabetes mellitus

Diabetes mellitus, the most common biochemical disease on the planet today, especially type 2 diabetes, is closely allied to obesity. Binge-eating being one of the primary drivers of obesity, therefore, occupies a special place in the list of risk factors for developing Non-insulin dependent

Diabetes Mellitus (NIDDM). Things are made worse by the fact that a large part of what you may be eating is going to be sugary. That only throws up a whole vista of other problems.

-Sleep disorders

Binge-eating can lead you towards the development of sleep disorders. First up is sleep apnea. The bigger you get due to BED, the harder it is going to be to keep your throat free while you sleep. Obese binge-eaters often have problems keeping their airways unblocked while they sleep, causing them to snore while they sleep and frequent breaks in sleep. On a psychological level, when you binge at night, it is quite possible for you to find it harder than usual to fall asleep no thanks to physical discomfort and the itch to consume more.

-Irritable Bowel Syndrome

IBS and other absorption disorders, such as ulcerative colitis, are more common in people with BED. Explanations have been inconclusive about why this is so, but what is sure is that as a binge-eater, you are more likely to have absorption disorders than the average individual out there.

-Substance abuse

One might ask how substance abuse can be a side effect of binge-eating, but it is. Depression and low esteem that follows BED around ensure that sufferers are never too far away from destructive implosions such as picking up substance abuse. The lure of substance and alcohol abuse to shore up the failing levels of esteem often trap many a binge-eater. Combined with excessive overeating, substance abuse further potentiates the self-destructive tendencies within binge-eaters.

Binge-eating, in its own right, serves as a genuine purveyor of various health, social and mental problems or people addicted to food. When it is closely allied to obesity, depression, and their attendant complications, the list of issues it brings triples and becomes almost endless.

# 13.Compulsive Eating Explained

There's often a misconception of compulsive eating and I aim to remove any misinterpretations of the condition. A variety of disorders exist and there are numerous warning signs to look out for if you're trying to help yourself or someone you care about. The comprehensive details on symptoms that accompany eating disorders will be expanded so that you can diagnose yourself with the malady because it's often difficult to recognize our faults.

## The Definition of Compulsive Eating

Where do we start when we're faced with a problem we deny? The beginning of this journey lies within recognizing what the problem is. You can't face an issue when you deny the existence of it. This remains true with every aspect of life. Someone who drinks alcoholic beverages excessively is often blinded by their perception. They develop tunnel vision and see no error in their decisions. They often cannot see the impact drinking has on their lives until it reaches astronomical significance and ravages their life to shreds. Just as alcohol impairs people, so does food and lifestyle. The food we consume is frequently overlooked, along with the snags it cultivates.

Life was so much simpler in ancient times. Heck, it was even effortless in the early 1900s. We weren't surrounded by endless temptations and food to console ourselves. What happened to the days where grass-fed animal and vegetable products were eaten as staple foods? Now we consume large laboratory-produced T-bone steaks at lunch and drown our cereal with refined sugar and pasteurized milk. We drink coffee out of habit and find solace in stuffing our faces when we're confronted with challenges in life. Come on, I know you've heard the phrase "comfort food" before. You know what I'm talking about. As humans, we have found comfort in eating to overcome the trials we meet. I'm not immune to this habit myself as I've succumbed to the same persuasion before. However, when I found out what defined this eating disorder, my vision changed, and I began looking for answers.

How does one describe compulsive eating? I want you to focus on the word "compulsive." The description which immediately comes to mind is revealing in itself. Compulsive means to have an irresistible urge which stems deep within you. Your urge overwhelms your senses and brain to create an irrefutable delusion. "Irresistible" is another keyword because you can't resist something that creates an overpowering desire inside of you. This influential impulse convinces you that what you desire is compulsory. It tricks your mind into altering a basic desire into something you strongly believe is needed for the likes of your survival and happiness. It becomes your only desire when you experience this impulse. Compulsive behavior is dangerous, to say the least.

When this impulse is combined with the vast array of foods, healthy and unhealthy, it explodes into a detrimental behavior of overeating. Compulsive overeating portrays itself as someone who consumes colossal amounts of food or calories that aren't perceived as normal. It doesn't necessarily mean the person eats their food in five minutes. Overeating or binge eating can also present itself as someone eating more food in two hours than someone else would eat over two or three meals throughout the day.

If you look at someone and their portion of food is substantially different from yours, it could indicate that you're overeating. In some cases, the portion may resemble yours in size but yours is smothered in gravy and three variants of sauces with a stack of fries that reach for the heavens. Ask yourself one question: Are you able to finish a large pack of potato chips and a jumbo soda in five minutes without feeling satisfied? Do you eat for flavor or is it an absolute necessity for you to finish your plate of food? Think about the last time you were so stuffed that you placed leftovers in the fridge for the following morning. There may be a problem if you can't remember a time you didn't finish your meal.

Nevertheless, compulsive eating is a behavior common in many serious eating disorders. It's not an eating disorder on its own but it's a behavior that accompanies potentially life-threatening eating disorders. It describes the action of eating uncontrollably and having no brakes. The person will find themselves eating until they become physically uncomfortable and their button is about to pop. They may continue eating until they become sick in some instances. They lose the ability to recognize when they're satisfied and fail to slam on the brakes on the train of consumption.

This behavioral disorder results in you feeling out of control in your own body. It can intensify to a point where regulation is long lost. Sufferers can be enticed to eat after smelling something delectable, even though they've just eaten. They become a zombie who's lost all impulse control and the mere sight, smell, and even audio stimuli can activate the cravings like a zombie craves the flesh of another person. Compulsive eating zombies might start eating to a point where their upper abdomen extends, and they experience pain in their lower chest from the pressure on their diaphragm.

Compulsive eating contains impulse control distortions. However, it also consists of obsession with food, weight, and physique. An obsession creates another insalubrious train smash with desire. Therefore, having a compulsive eating distortion can be defined as having an obsession too.

## Common Symptoms

I know that I've touched a nerve here and you want to know more. You might have suffered the same chain of events I did before you reached obesity. Nevertheless, there are symptoms associated with compulsive overeating and some of them can indicate a specific disorder. I'm going to guide you through identifying worrisome symptoms, but an accurate diagnosis should be specified by a doctor, nutrition specialist, or a therapist. I aim to help someone who suffers from compulsive overeating in general and my advice will pertain to that.

Typical symptoms tied to compulsive overeating, in general, include a variety of tell-tale signs. If you can relate to even one or two of these signs, you're most likely suffering from this impulsive alien. Someone who overeats impulsively will eat amounts that are larger than what someone else would consider rational. They could eat at a speed which puts Michael Schumacher to shame (Schumacher is a retired formula one driver who was contracted by the likes of Ferrari). On the other hand, you could eat at the speed in which David Hasselhoff moves in his infamous slow-motion Baywatch program. Unfortunately, people who eat with persistent buffering can result in never finding an end. They commonly eat non-stop throughout the day.

Eating until their bubble is about to burst is another easily identifiable symptom. They eat past a state of suffice and frequently indulge in consumption when they're not even hungry. They could begin eating out of boredom or to soothe any emotional disturbance. Feelings of guilt and shame drive them to eat alone because they're afraid of judgment on the size of their portion or embarrassed by their manner of consumption. They inevitably feel guilty, depressed, and even disgusted in themselves after binge eating. They find themselves divulging in the temptation in the middle of the night when the world is asleep. The most frightening tribute is when they begin hiding their food or eating in secrecy.

In 1999, there was a movie called The Spy Who Shagged Me and it starred Mike Myers as Austin Powers. It was a huge hit and I personally loved the Austin Powers movies, as corny as they were. However, Myers doubled as another character in this specific rendition who tugs at my heartstrings. The character was called "fat bastard" for comedic purposes but one line from the movie is true. Fat bastard lies on the bed, in his sumo outfit, indulging in food, and says, "I eat because I'm sad and I'm sad because I eat." There's an undeniable truth in his words and another symptom you can identify eating disorders with is the irrefutable connection between your emotions and eating. Someone who impulsively divulges in excessive amounts of food will become depressed about their obsession and, in turn, the depression will worsen the problem. Look out for these signs as well because they play a large role in your behavior. The bottom line is that emotional distress after eating a meal is a definite sign of consumption issues.

Someone who suffers from BED may feel out of control when they eat. The second symptom is when someone excessively overeats and has no accountability for their behavior. They recognize a problem, but they don't care about the consequences. They use no form of purging to supplement their behavior and go about life gaining weight and increasing the risk to their health. Don't get me wrong, purging is extremely dangerous to your health as well.

When it comes to bulimia nervosa, there's also no perceived ability to regulate their actions and a sense of ill management exists. Additional symptoms can include a severe fear of gaining weight even though their body mass index is normal, a brutally impaired self-esteem about themselves, and purging.

You may be embracing a corrupt eating habit if any of the symptoms are prevalent at least once a week for three months or more. If you're experiencing these symptoms like a new addition to your life, you should step up immediately. The sooner you correct the problem, the easier the task will be. The good news is that overeaters are usually aware of their symptoms and that itself is another symptom. They acknowledge that their eating habits are abnormal.

# 14.The Power of Repeated Words and Thoughts

Experts estimate that an average adult experiences sixty thousand thoughts in a day. Fifty thousand of these are negative. A whopping eighty percent of our thoughts are negative and unproductive. Repetitive negative thoughts can cause illness and negative outcomes in our lives. Words have a remarkable effect on our lives. They provide us with a means to share our selves and our life experiences with others. The words we regularly use affect the experiences we have in our lives. By switching up your vocabulary, you can switch up your life.

Repetition is a powerful learning tool as it is known as the "mother" of all learning. Hypnotherapists utilize repetition wisely to pack on all aspects of hypnosis. That is the same reason that relaxes the mind during repetitive hypnosis. It is said that if something frequently happens to a desired degree or amount, you will be persuaded. That is why adverts will play consistently and on repeat because repetition is about creating a familiar pattern in abundance. When you experience something over and over again, the mind understands the phenomena causing the experience to become lodged in your memory. It is repeated so many times that it becomes convincing and to some extent, nagging. Like when a chewing gum song will not leave your mind, and you keep repeating it all day long.

Repetitive thought has made its way into our lives through many channels. Remember the Lord's Prayer? We can recite it by heart because it was pounded in us at an early age. So were nursery rhymes like "Row your boat." Repetition is present in songs, musical notes, prayers, chants, mantras, and many other forms of literary works. We assign weight and importance to our thoughts to determine which ones stay longer in our minds. Repetition is often reacted to as a social cue from a colleague. When people witness something done repetitively, they too begin to do it. That is how social media has become the plague it is.

When emotions are linked to certain things, repetition can be used as a trigger to awaken those emotions. The hypnotic triple is a hypnosis rule of thumb in some schools that states that something is suggested three times to culminate an effect. Not merely saying the words thrice, but also including the theme and any emotion that may be associated with it. The mind enjoys repetition because it is calming, and calming is always good. Therefore, reconstructing your subconscious mind to have dominant positive beliefs, thoughts, and habits, the more favorable your outlook on life will be.

## Repetition and the Subconscious Mind

Your subconscious mind is impartial, unrelenting, and faithful. It does most of the sifting through all of our thoughts and relates them with our senses then communicates with the conscious mind through emotions. The subconscious mind collects your thoughts and stimuli from your environment and works on forming reactions to it. For example, you may see a particular person, perhaps your neighbor and feel dislike; you may even form a scowl. Yet, you have never exchanged three words with your neighbor. Why do you feel like this towards him/her? The information you fed your subconscious. The illusory truth effect is a phenomenon where something arbitrary becomes true because it was repeated over and over again when no one was paying any attention to it.

However, we do not know what the unconscious mind is working on because it does its works "behind the scenes." We cannot "sense" it hard at work, nor can we stop its processes. The good news then is that you can feed your mind with certain notions and ideals to elicit the emotions you have associated with them. Do not think, however, that the subconscious mind listens to reason; remember it remains an impartial participant in your everyday life. Take an example and remember when you tried to reason with an irrational phobia- of heights or tight spaces- for example. The conscious mind knows for a fact that there is nothing to fear, but you cannot help reacting in a particular way to these fears like getting sick, for example, and feeling dizzy.

Therefore, because your subconscious mind goes in the direction you command it; if you repeatedly affirm positive thoughts such as "I am beautiful," or "I can do this," you will automatically begin to develop a different attitude towards yourself. You will develop an inner outlook of your life which will gingerly propel you toward recognizing and taking advantage of the opportunities that come knocking at your door. The conscious mind can willingly train the subconscious mind and test the outcome using your life experiences. An excellent example of this is the power of autosuggestion. Have you heard of a vision board? They are ideas or fantasies that you pin up on a board that is strategically placed near the eye line. The more you repeatedly see the board, the more information you are giving the subconscious mind. After a while, check to see if there are any notable improvements in your life. For most people, it takes roughly three months to see some progress, depending on how powerful your autosuggestions are.

## Affirmations and Belief

Beliefs are formed by repetitive thought that has been nourished over and over for an extended period. Affirmations are positively charged proclamations or pronouncements repeated severally through the day, every day. These words are often terse, straightforward, memorable, and repetitive. Affirmations are phrased in the present tense and they lead to belief. The most crucial element of any self-improvement process is to set an intention. Muhammud Ali once said that "It is the repetition of affirmations that cause belief, and when the beliefs become deep convictions, that is when things start to happen."

Let's say you intend to shed some weight. That being the sole goal, it is paramount that all your efforts are focused on achieving it. Therefore, affirmative statements should be in the lines of, "Shedding pounds is as easy as packing them on," "I am what I eat," "A healthy mind is a healthy body," "I feel beautiful on the outside as I do on the inside," and so on. Keep in mind that not all the words you utter will yield results. For affirmations to work, they have to be coupled with visualization and a feeling of conviction. Therefore, it is advisable to focus more on positive thoughts than negative thoughts and for a prolonged period.

Remember to use words that resonate with you. The affirmations need not be empty for you. They ought to have a close relation and meaning attached to them. The proper statements for the appropriate situation go a long way in achieving success.

You can try repeating your affirmations before you go to bed. As the brain gets ready to go on "autopilot" mode, the subconscious mind becomes more active, thereby absorbing the last bits of information for the day. Repeating affirmations before you sleep not only makes you slip into dreamland in a more confident and relaxed state but also helps to convince the mind.

You might begin to wonder why, if affirmations work, they are not used to get out of "tricky" situations. For example, if you are feeling sick, would you proceed to state, "I am cured. I am well,"? Affirmations work best with an aligned state of mind. If you believe to be well, it is more likely that you will begin to notice a decline in symptoms. If you do not believe in your affirmations, you will continue to battle through the temperature and other physical discomforts.

Finding the right words to use can be a stroll in the park; however, remembering to repeat these words, severally could present itself as a challenge. The other obstacle you might face is having two conflicting thoughts. One of them is the carefully considered affirmation, while the other is a counterproductive negation. Try the best you can to disprove the negative thoughts but do not feed them time nor energy. It will be quite challenging to believe affirmations too at the beginning. However, as time goes on, it will become easier to convince yourself. Practice makes perfect.

Affirmations seem to work because:

- The act of repeating positive statements anchors your thoughts and energy, driving you toward their fulfillment
- Affirmations program the subconscious mind, which in turn processes your reactions to circumstances.
- The more frequently you repeat the affirmations, you become more attuned with your environment. You start seeing new opportunities, and your mind opens up to new ways of fulfilling your goals

## Repetition and Hypnosis

Hypnosis aims at the subconscious part of our minds to elicit lasting behavioral changes. As we have already established, repetition relaxes the mind, and when it is employed in hypnosis, the patient arrives at a state of extreme relaxation. Hypnotic suggestions can yield positive outcomes provided the intentions are set. There are two techniques used to harness the power of repetition in hypnosis.

## Listen then Repeat

To bring about success during hypnosis, you must be a good listener. When someone is speaking to you, listen cautiously to both their verbal and non-verbal cues. See what both their conscious and subconscious minds are telling you. If possible, note them down.

Then say it back to them. Repeat their suggestions back to them in the language they used. When you say something in a similar tone and style, the person tends to take it as "The Gospel." Notwithstanding they feel heard and find their thoughts acceptable when they are repeated. For example, if someone says to you "I want to shed some weight to feel more like myself," you may report back to them, "You have shed some weight, and you are feeling more like yourself." Suppose you said, "You are thin, and you are feeling more like yourself." That suggestion would be utterly useless because the language used was different, therefore ineffective.

## Repetitive Themes

Because themes can mean different things to different people, they become a powerful suggestive tool. Let's say a specific client always talks about one particular direction in all the meetings. Losing weight and becoming more of themselves, for instance. Take the recurrent theme and run with it. The best hypnotherapists deliver the same piece of information is a variety of ways through repetition to reinforce the principle.

You can use repetitive themes to formulate smart suggestions that are more powerful. If the subject is narrow and too specific, allow your client to broaden the topic and use the information to generalize their theme.

When appropriately applied, both techniques offer simplicity and effectiveness because hypnotherapy patients have the solutions within themselves, not to mention the brain is soothed by repetition. Therefore, the power of personal suggestion is comfortable and safe.

## Using Affirmations During Self-hypnosis

It is important to reiterate that set and setting are of paramount concern. That means that it is advisable to conduct self-hypnosis in an environment where you are not likely to be disturbed- not while operating machinery or working. Let the people in your proximity know that you will be taking a nap (because hypnosis is much like falling asleep- except with heightened sensitivity) this way; you will not be interrupted.

Step 1: Write Your Script

Ensure that the text includes the beginning that is the relaxation technique. Here, you will add the repetitive sounds and if possible, visions of the ocean, if you love the ocean waves, or the sound of falling rain, or perhaps the forest. This element will relax you, and you will begin to feel physically relaxed and comfortable.

While you are in the relaxed space, repeat your affirmations about ten to fifteen times with natural deep breaths between each mantra. Continue enjoying the comfortable space you are in, taking in the smells, sights, sounds, and temperature. As you draw in all the senses from the space you are in, add to them the emotions triggered that particular "safe" space. As you start to feel, repeat the affirmations one more time. The conclusion of your script should include a dissociation between the trance state and the reality.

Step 2: Record Your Script

Talk slowly into the recording device. Slow your pace and remember your intention for doing this. The result will be more impactful if you slow your roll and allow the subconscious mind to absorb the words as you say them. The affirmations should include statements like, "I am 10-pounds lighter," "I have control over my body," and the like.

Step 3: Find a Quiet, Comfortable Space Where You Will Remain Uninterrupted for a Few Minutes

Keep in mind that when you are attempting a hypnotherapy session, the body temperature tends to fall below average. You can prepare for this using blankets or warm clothing. Put on your earpieces and listen to your recording.

Become aware of your eyelids getting heavier, and heavier as you gradually close your eyes. Remember to maintain a steady breathing motion- not too fast, not too slow. The breaths should be natural, do not struggle or pant for air. With every breath, feel yourself becoming more relaxed.

All the while keeps your mind's eye focused on the repetitive swing of the pendulum. Count slowly downwards. Start from a comfortable number, perhaps eight or ten and with each number take a deep breath into relaxation. Believe that when you finish the countdown, you will have arrived at your ideal trance state. Once you arrive, it is time to pay attention to your affirmations.

Step 4: Listen to the Recording Every Day

Commitment is key. As you listen to your affirmations, make sure to repeat them.

It is also necessary to clear your mind before attempting to get into a hypnotic state. There are several ways of clearing the mind; for example, in the advent of hypnosis, a pendulum was used to draw the attention of the mind and maintain it. The repetitive motion of the swing causes the mind to slip into a trance state. The more you repeat the process of self-hypnosis, the easier it will become for you to reach a hypnotic state, and successfully alter your life.

The law of repetition states that repetition of behavior causes it to be more potent as each suggestion acted upon creates less opposition for the following suggestions. If you are looking to change your habits, it is of uttermost importance that you are prepared to put in the work. Reprogramming the mind towards more real life-fulfilling goals can be an uphill climb because when habits form, they become harder to break and more comfortable to follow for all organs involved. However, all of that is learned in muscle memory. That is why repetition is emphasized. Meaning that because the mind is a muscle, it can be trained to take in more information, or rewrite existing knowledge. Just like the gym, it requires a commitment to see the results. As you practice repetition frequently, maintain actionable momentum on the subconscious and conscious levels of learning. Repetition is how successes are created.

# 15.Affirmation to Cut Calories

Affirmations are a wonderful tool to use alongside hypnosis to help you rewire your brain and improve your weight loss abilities. Affirmations are essentially a tool that you use to remind you of your chosen "rewiring" and to encourage your brain to opt for your newer, healthier mindset over your old unhealthy one. Using affirmations is an important part of anchoring your hypnosis efforts into your daily life, so it is important that you use them on a routine basis.

When using affirmations, it is important that you use ones that are relevant and that are going to actually support you in anchoring your chosen reality into your present reality.

## What Are Affirmations, and How Do They Work?

Anytime you repeat something to yourself out loud, or in your thoughts, you are affirming something to yourself. We use affirmations on a consistent basis, whether we consciously realize it or not. For example, if you are on your weight loss journey and you repeat "I am never going to lose the weight" to yourself on a regular basis, you are affirming to yourself that you are never going to succeed with weight loss. Likewise, if you are consistently saying, "I will always be fat" or "I am never going to reach my goals" you are affirming those things to yourself, too.

When we use affirmations unintentionally, we often find ourselves using affirmations that can be hurtful and harmful to our psyche and our reality. You might find yourself locking into becoming a mental bully toward yourself as you consistently repeat things to yourself that are unkind and even downright mean. As you do this, you affirm a lower sense of self-confidence, a lack of motivation, and a commitment to a body shape and wellness journey that you do not actually want to maintain.

Affirmations, whether positive or negative, conscious, or unconscious, are always creating or reinforcing the function of your brain and mindset. Each time you repeat something to yourself, your subconscious mind hears it and strives to make it a part of your reality. This is because your subconscious mind is responsible for creating your reality and your sense of identity. It creates both around your affirmations since these are what you perceive as being your absolute truth; therefore, they create a "concrete" foundation for your reality and identity to rest on. If you want to change these two aspects of yourself and your experience, you are going to need to change what you are routinely repeating to yourself so that you are no longer creating a reality and identity rooted in negativity.

In order to change your subconscious experience, you need to consciously choose positive affirmations and repeat them on a constant basis to help you achieve the reality and identity that you truly want. This way, you are more likely to create an experience that reflects what you are looking for, rather than an experience that reflects what your conscious and subconscious mind has automatically picked up on.

The key with affirmations is that you need to understand that your brain does not care if you are creating them on purpose or not. It also does not care if you are creating healthy and positive ones or unhealthy and negative ones. All your subconscious mind cares about is what is repeated to it, and what you perceive as being your absolute truth. It is up to you and your conscious mind to recognize that negative and unhealthy affirmations will hold you back, prevent you from experiencing positive experiences in life, and result in you feeling incapable and unmotivated. Alternatively, consciously choosing healthy and positive affirmations will help you with creating a mindset that is healthier and an identity that actually serves your wellbeing on a mental, physical, emotional, and spiritual level. From there, your responsibility is to consistently repeat these affirmations to yourself until you believe them, and you begin to see them being reflected in your reality.

## How Do I Pick and Use Affirmations for Weight Loss?

Choosing affirmations for your weight loss journey requires you to first understand what it is that you are looking for, and what types of positive thoughts are going to help you get there. You can start by identifying what your dream is, what you want your ideal body to look and feel like, and how you want to feel as you achieve your dream of losing weight. Once you have identified what your dream is, you need to identify what current beliefs you have around the dream that you are aspiring to achieve. For example, if you want to lose 25 pounds so that you can have a healthier weight, but you believe that it will be incredibly hard to lose that weight, then you know that your current beliefs are that losing weight is hard. You need to identify every single belief surrounding your weight loss goals and recognize which ones are negative or are limiting and preventing you from achieving your goal of losing weight.

After you have identified which of your beliefs are negative and unhelpful, you can choose affirmations that are going to help you change your beliefs. Typically, you want to choose an affirmation that is going to help you completely change that belief in the opposite direction. For example, if you think "losing weight is hard," your new affirmation could be "I lose the weight effortlessly." Even if you do not believe this new affirmation right now, the goal is to repeat it to yourself enough that it becomes a part of your identity and, inevitably, your reality. This way, you are anchoring in your hypnosis sessions, and you are effectively rewiring your brain in between sessions, too.

As you use affirmations to help you achieve weight loss, I encourage you to do so in a way that is intuitive to your experience. There is no right or wrong way to approach affirmations, as long as you are using them on a regular basis. Once you feel yourself effortlessly believing in an affirmation, you can start incorporating new affirmations into your routine so that you can continue to use your affirmations to improve your wellbeing overall. Ideally, you should always be using positive affirmations even after you have seen the changes you desire, as affirmations are a wonderful way to help naturally maintain your mental, emotional, and physical wellbeing.

## What Should I Do with My Affirmations?

After you have chosen what affirmations you want to use, and which ones are going to feel best for you, you need to know what to do with them! The simplest way to use your affirmations is to pick 1-2 affirmations and repeat them to yourself on a regular basis. You can repeat them anytime you feel the need to re-affirm something to yourself, or you can repeat them continually even if they do not seem entirely relevant in the moment. The key is to make sure that you are always repeating them to yourself so that you are more likely to have success in rewiring your brain and achieving the new, healthier, and more effective beliefs that you need to improve the quality of your life.

In addition to repeating your affirmations to yourself, you can also use them in many other ways. One way that people like using affirmations is by writing them down. You can write your affirmations down on little notes and leave them around your house, or you can make a ritual out of writing your affirmations down a certain amount of times per day in a journal so that you are able to routinely work them into your day. Some people will also meditate on their affirmations, meaning that they essentially meditate and then repeat the affirmations to themselves over and over in a meditative state. If repeating your affirmation to yourself like a mantra is too challenging, you can also say your chosen affirmations to yourself on a voice recording track and then repeat them to yourself on loop while you meditate. Other people will create recordings of themselves repeating several affirmations into their voice recorder and then listening to them on loop while they work out, eat, drive to work, or otherwise engage in an activity where affirmations might be useful.

If you really want to make your affirmations effective and get the most out of them, you need to find a way to essentially bombard your brain with this new information. The more effectively you can do this, the more your subconscious brain is going to pick up on it and continue to reinforce your new neural pathways with these new affirmations. Through that, you will find yourself effortlessly and naturally believing in the new affirmations that you have chosen for yourself.

## How Are Affirmations Going to Help Me Lose Weight?

Affirmations are going to help you lose weight in a few different ways. First and foremost, and probably most obvious, is the fact that affirmations are going to help you get in the mindset of weight loss. To put it simply: you cannot sit around believing nothing is going to work and expect things to work for you. You need to be able to cultivate a motivated mindset that allows you to create success. If you are unable to believe that it will come true: trust that it will not come true.

As your mindset improves, your subconscious mind is actually going to start changing other things within your body, too. For example, rather than creating desires and cravings for things that are not healthy for you, your body will begin to create desires and cravings for things that are healthy for you. It will also stop creating inner conflict around making the right choices and taking care of yourself. In fact, you may even find yourself actually falling in love with your new diet and your new exercise routine. You will also likely find yourself naturally leaning toward behaviors and habits that are healthier for you without having to try so hard to create those habits. In many cases, you might create habits that are healthy for you without even realizing that you are creating those habits. Rather than having to consciously become aware of the need for habits, and then putting in the work to create them, your body and mind will naturally begin to recognize the need for better habits and will create those habits naturally as well.

Some studies have also suggested that using affirmations will help your brain and subconscious mind actually govern your body differently, too. For example, you may be able to improve your body's ability to digest things and manage your weight naturally by using affirmations and hypnosis. In doing so, you may be able to subconsciously adjust which hormones, chemicals, and enzymes are created within your body to help with things like digestive functions, energy creation, and other weight- and health-related concerns that you may have.

## Affirmations for Self-Control

Self-control is an important discipline to have, and not having it can lead to behaviors that are known for making weight loss more challenging. If you are struggling with self-control, the following affirmations will help you change any beliefs you have around self-control so that you can start approaching food, exercise, weight loss, and wellness in general with healthier beliefs.

1. I have self-control.
2. My willpower is my superpower.
3. I am in complete control of myself in this experience.
4. I make my own choices.
5. I have the power to decide.
6. I am dedicated to achieving my goals.
7. I will make the best choice for me.
8. I succeed because I have self-control.
9. I am capable of working through hardships.
10. I am dedicated to overcoming challenges.
11. My mind is strong, powerful, and disciplined.
12. I am in control of my desires.

13. My mindset is one of success.
14. I become more disciplined every day.
15. Self-discipline comes easily for me.
16. Self-control comes easily for me.
17. I achieve success because I am in control.
18. I find it easier to succeed every day.
19. I see myself as a successful, self-disciplined person.
20. Self-control comes effortlessly for me.
21. Self-control is as natural as breathing.
22. I have control over my thoughts.
23. I have control over my choices.
24. I can trust my willpower to carry me through.
25. I can tap into self-control whenever I need to.
26. My self-control is stronger than my desire.
27. I am incredibly strong with self-control.
28. I easily maintain my self-control in all situations.
29. I see things through to the end.
30. I can depend on myself to make healthy choices.
31. Healthy choices are easy for me to make.
32. It is easy for me to control my impulses.
33. Self-control is my natural state.
34. I will keep going until I reach my goal.
35. I am starting to love the feeling of self-control.

36. I see myself as a successful person.
37. I have unbreakable willpower.
38. I have excellent self-control.
39. I am a highly self-disciplined person.
40. I succeed with every goal I create.
41. I am a highly intentional person.
42. Every day, my self-control gets stronger.
43. I am becoming highly disciplined.
44. I am successful because of my self-discipline.
45. I am a strong, capable person.
46. I am dedicated to achieving my wellness goals.
47. Self-control is one of my greatest strengths.
48. I am in complete control of this situation.
49. I can do this.
50. I am self-aware and capable.
51. I can move forward with self-control and gratitude.
52. I always do what I say I am going to do.
53. I show up as my best self, and I achieve my dreams.
54. I have the willpower to make this happen.
55. I can count on myself to make the right choice.
56. I trust my strength to carry me through.
57. I am becoming stronger every day.
58. I make my choices with self-discipline.

59. I have the discipline to see this through.
60. I make my choices intentionally.
61. I am committed to my success.

## Affirmations for Exercise

Exercise is necessary for healthy weight loss, but it can be challenging to commit to. Many people struggle with motivating themselves to exercise, or to exercise enough, to take proper care of their body. If you are struggling with exercising, these affirmations will help motivate you to work out or motivate you to finish your workout on a high note.

1. I am so excited to exercise.
2. I love moving my body.
3. I am focused and ready to exercise.
4. I am showing up at 100%.
5. Today, I will have an excellent workout.
6. I have the courage to see this workout through.
7. My body is becoming stronger every day.
8. I love exercising.
9. Exercising is fun and exciting.
10. I love becoming the best version of myself.
11. Exercising is one of my favorite activities.
12. Exercising makes me feel happy and healthy.
13. I have a strong body and mind.
14. I am confident about my ability to see this through.
15. I can feel myself becoming stronger.

16. I can feel myself becoming leaner.
17. My body is getting healthier every single day.
18. I am transforming my body every day.
19. I am creating the body I have always wanted.
20. Every day I am losing weight.
21. I am getting thinner every single day.
22. Each day I get closer to my ideal weight.
23. I am motivated to take care of my body.
24. I am excited to lose weight in a healthy, natural way.
25. My body is capable of being healthy.
26. I love how flexible my body is becoming.
27. Maintaining my ideal weight is as easy as breathing.
28. My weight is dropping quickly and in a healthy way.
29. I am dedicated to having a stronger body.
30. I feel myself getting stronger every single day.
31. My body deserves a healthy workout.
32. I love creating my dream body.
33. Having a strong body is important to me.
34. I am motivated to reach my fitness goals.
35. I am determined to have a healthier body.
36. I am so proud of myself for my growth.
37. I am strong and motivated.
38. I am committed to having a healthier body.

39. I easily become motivated to exercise.

40. I am capable of having a healthier body.

# 16.Low of Attraction

Your thoughts can be used for good or bad without even realizing it. Unfortunately, most of what we see and hear today is negative. News, media, music, coworkers, and even family members can spread negative thoughts with no direct intention. When our minds are taking in negative information, that becomes our thoughts and our thoughts become our actions.

Scientists tell us that our thoughts generate unique frequencies that attract back to us like frequencies. This is known as the Law of Attraction. This universal law states that we generate the things, events, and people that appear in our lives. Our thoughts, feelings, words, and actions produce energies (unique frequency) that attract like energies. Negative energies attract negative energies and positive energies attract positive energies.

This means nothing happens in our lives by coincidence. You attract everything into your life, everything that happens to you, through your thoughts, feelings, words, and actions. Notice that this chain of events begins with your thoughts. Knowing this will make it easier to understand why having negative thoughts of depression, anger, hatred, greed, or selfishness to name a few, can bring you more of the same.

By learning to directly control your thoughts, you are able to block out negative energies. This can be accomplished by thinking only positive thoughts. Positive thinking is a theory that many ancient masters and philosophers have used throughout history.

Successful men and women have used positive thinking to inspire thousands. Many teachers and motivational speakers today use the power of positive thinking to help change people's lives for the better. This positive thinking technique is easier said than done however.

To think positively you have to concentrate on your thoughts, especially at first. The minute your subconscious mind takes over, it can fall back into old habits of negative thinking. Practicing to think positive all day long will take some effort considering we have 35-48 thoughts per minute. Being persistent in regard to thinking positively will eventually become a habit and a new way of life.

You will start to notice good things happening to you. You'll notice things seem to fall into place and go your way. Do not dismiss this phenomenon as a mere coincidence. It is great powers at work. The more evidence you obtain that it's working, the easier it will become to master. Before you know it, you'll be living the life you've always dreamed of. A life of success and happiness anyone would appreciate.

Most people underestimate the power of their thoughts. They think that thought is nothing, that thoughts are not things, and therefore that they cannot affect reality. Science has already shown that this is not true, our ways of thinking determine most of the things that happen to us, we just don't realize it. You can easily see it paying attention to the little everyday things, for example how a thought, an emotion or a state of mind instantly influence your physiology and your body.

Think about when you are afraid; the thought of something that scares you can increase sweating, accelerate the heartbeat and breathing. In the same way, even the less important sensations for survival, like a positive emotion, can have real physical effects.

Think for example when you listen to a song that you like or that gives you intense emotions, it is not a mere sensation that stops only in the mind, it spreads like a wave in the whole body, some people, for example, get goosebumps ... This means that thought has had a physical, real and tangible effect on their body and their physiology.

Thoughts have the power not only directly on you, but they shape the reality in which you live. A positive thought attracts positive things and shifts your focus to positive events, it is a bit like when you are driving and you are late, you will find many more red lights on your path, in reality you are the one who puts the focus on the obstacles, so you notice much more negative things and you feel therefore unlucky, which increases your attention even more in noticing negative things, thus creating a destructive spiral. Remember, anything you focus on, will grow.

Then, the regular and constant repetition over time of positive affirmations can reprogram our brain on a positive mindset, and creates a virtuous circle in which we begin to notice more positive things and consequently leads us to receive them in greater quantity, creating an infinite loop of gratitude and attraction of the good.

Your faith and your love are energy, which, by interacting with the energy of the universe, will attract to you everything you want strongly.

The affirmations you are about to hear, if repeated a sufficient number of times, will become rooted in your unconscious and will replace the negative paradigms you may have developed from your childhood until today. This process will change the lenses through which you look at the world and your life will turn into something wonderful and unique, making you grateful and able to appreciate all the things you have and will attract.

The Law of Attraction is not a new concept. It's always been around and it's constantly working, whether you believe in it or not. You can't get better at using the Law of Attraction because you're already using it. It already does work perfectly, 100% of the time. Practical Law of Attraction helps you get better at getting into alignment with the manifesting conditions, so you can manifest your heart's desire.

Perhaps you've heard it defined as "ask, believe, and achieve," or some other 3-step process.

These featured steps are important elements to manifesting. However, it goes way deeper than that. What about action? When they say "believe," are they saying consciously or unconsciously?

Certainly, if you focus on those three steps, it's possible you might get results. However, if you are getting results focusing on only those three steps, then it's because you are unconsciously also applying some unmentioned steps.

If you haven't been getting results, then you'll understand why as we go through the manifesting conditions.

## Here's How I Define Law of Attraction:

"Law of Attraction is when the manifesting conditions and personal qualities are developed and come into alignment simultaneously."

It's an impersonal law. It's unbiased. In other words, it doesn't matter if what you think, imagine, feel, or believe is something you fear or something you desire, the law works the same exact way—always. It simply manifests whatever you are in alignment with.

Law of Attraction is not a quick fix. It is a way of life.

It's not a step by step formula or process, because you are starting "the process" from where you are right now, your own unique set of circumstances.

As you explore each of the manifesting conditions, you will gain a better understanding of how you have created the life situation, you're in now. You'll also learn the ways to stop creating more unwanted circumstances, and ultimately create a life you truly love.

## How did Law of Attraction Originate?

The New Thought movement grew out of the teachings of Phineas Quimby in the early 19th Century. Early in his life, Quimby was diagnosed with tuberculosis. Unfortunately, medicinal treatment wasn't working.

In 1838, Quimby began studying Mesmerism. He became aware of the mental and placebo effect of the mind over the body when prescribed medicines of no physical value cured patients of diseases. From there, Phineas Quimby developed theories of mentally aided healing

It wasn't until 1877 that the term "Law of Attraction" first appeared in print, in a book which discusses esoteric mysteries of ancient theosophy, called Isis Unveiled, written by the Russian occultist, Helena Blavatsky, where she alluded to an attractive power existing between elements of spirit.

However, there have been many references even before the term was used, that describe what we understand today.

Gautama Buddha, (who lived between 563 BC - 480 BC): said "What we are today comes from our thoughts of yesterday, and our present thoughts build our life of tomorrow: Our life is the creation of our mind."

Empedocles (490 BC), an early Greek philosopher, hypothesized something called Love (philia) to explain the attraction of different forms of matter.

Plato alleged as early as (391 BC): "Like tends towards like."

The Bible has many statements suggesting the power of having faith and asking for what you want, such as: "Ask, and it shall be given you; seek, and ye shall find; knock and it shall be opened unto you."

By the 20th Century, a surge in interest in the subject led to many books being written about it, including:

The Science of Getting Rich (1910) by Wallace D. Wattles

The Master Key System (1912) Charles Haanel

How to Win Friends and Influence People (1936) Dale Carnegie

Think and Grow Rich (1937) Napoleon Hill

The Power of Positive Thinking (1952) Norman Vincent Peale

The Power of Your Subconscious Mind (1962) Joseph Murphy

Creative Visualization (1978) Shakti Gawain

You Can Heal Your Life (1980) Louise Hay

Law of Intention and Desire (1994) Deepak Chopra

How to Get What You Really, Really, Really, Really Want (1998) Wayne Dyer, public television special

The Secret (2006): The concept of the Law of Attraction gained a lot of renewed exposure with the release of the film and book written by Rhonda Byrne.

Since then, Law of Attraction became a bit more well-known. However, since the film represents the topic in a very basic manner with an inadequate basis for real-world application it contributes to some skepticism.

## Things that Aren't True

Myth #1: The Law of Attraction Isn't True

It always surprises me how many bright, intelligent people there are who learn about Law of Attraction and flippantly write it off as nonsense. The only issue with Law of Attraction is one of misunderstanding of what it is and how it works.

Before you dismiss the Law of Attraction, ask yourself this: Would aligning your thoughts, feelings, beliefs, and behaviors with what you want help you or hinder you?

Here's the thing, a belief in the Law of Attraction is a belief in your ability to have control over deliberately creating your reality and manifesting whatever you desire.

The idea you have a say in how your life is going infuriates some people. I can only assume this is because they are receiving some counter intentions by remaining stuck in a belief system that supports them in maintaining a victim mentality.

If you are of the opinion that what you think and feel has no bearing on your reality, you will not be able to attract results that you desire.

The mind is set up in such a way that it favors information that conforms to your existing beliefs and discounts evidence that does not.

Remember, the Law of Attraction is always working. How it works for you is up to you.

Myth #2: The Law of Attraction Is Like a Genie Granting Your Every Wish

This is the myth which continues to perpetuate Myth #1, that it doesn't work. Since Law of Attraction does not actually work like a genie, those who go into it thinking all they need to do is make a wish and a magic genie will miraculously appear and grant their heart's desire are setting themselves up for disillusionment.

Approaching Law of Attraction, coming from this idea you can think yourself into receiving high-ticket items, like cars, dream homes, and lottery winnings, and change your life overnight, is unhealthy. It is the very reason why critics, skepticism, and misunderstanding about this Law exist.

While it's possible to achieve what you desire, it's going to require much more than thinking. It takes diligent effort to grow yourself into the person who is in alignment with your true desires.

Law of Attraction is common sense. It's a set of practical conditions the most successful people are naturally in alignment with. You need to have a clear desire and intention. Focus is required. You also need to be intentionally taking actions toward achieving what you want to create.

The more you align yourself with these conditions, the more the universal creative energy corresponds by sending you new ideas, intuitive messages, opportunities, helpful people, and other resources.

Myth #3: When Bad Stuff Happens, it is All Your Fault

No one knows exactly why catastrophic, horrible events happen to innocent, good, and well-intentioned people.

Some Law of Attraction advocates go too far and say you are responsible for every bad thing that's ever happened to you. There are no good answers to why terrible events happen to good people. I'm talking about the likes of getting raped, having your home burn down to the ground, or learning that you or a loved-one has been diagnosed with a terminal illness.

You certainly have every right to feel and process all the emotions you undergo when you experience a devastating loss or tragedy. One reason people remain stuck from moving on is they did not process their feelings. You can only heal what you feel.

The Law of Attraction is not about blaming you for everything that's ever happened to you in your life. Understand that sometimes bad things happen, like losing your job, going through a bad break-up, or not getting approved for your loan. Often enough, you can look back on those situations and see something better happened as a result, and it never would have happened had the bad thing never occurred.

What if, when bad things happened, you were to remain open to discovering how the event might play into a much grander, more intelligent plan that the universe has in store for you?

Here are a few other theories about why negative things might happen and how to deal with them when they do.

- The truth is, sometimes we do attract scenarios to ourselves by having fears about those things happening. Negative thoughts and energies do attract negative.

- If you believe in the concept that your soul has lived lives before this one, then you may be experiencing karma that originated several lifetimes ago.
- Again, if you believe in this idea that we have many lives and we create our lesson plans between lives, sometimes we orchestrate events we need to experience in this life for our soul to advance.
- It's completely random and we just don't have control over everything that happens to us. But we do have complete control over how we allow it to affect us as we navigate through our future.

The bottom line is, regardless of which scenario you subscribe to, it's tiresome and painful to try and pinpoint exactly why things happen to us. When life becomes difficult and painful, you have two options. 1) You can accept what happened; or 2) you can suffer.

Acceptance does not mean you are making the situation right or you like or want what happened. It simply means you have accepted the idea that no matter how much you dwell on it, you are not going to change what happened. Acceptance is a way of letting it go so you can make room for better things to happen.

One of the laws of nature is change or impermanence. The one constant is change. Everything and everyone will eventually die.

Make peace with the past. Accept it. Forgive it. Live in the present. Whatever happened, happened. Life is not always fair. If you are always focusing on how things were, and the injustice you feel, then you will continue to re-create your future from that state. No matter how bad it was, it is not happening now. It only exists in your memory. You do not have to let it control your thoughts, emotions, or bring it into your future.

Focus on what you have control over, which is how you choose to experience this present moment. Whatever you are focusing on, feeling, and imagining right now is what's creating your future.

## The Laws

## Universal Laws

Universal Laws are guidelines that help us understand the rules we are playing by.

Everything in the world is made of energy and we are all connected with that energy.

Our thoughts, feelings, words, and actions are all forms of energy and is what creates our reality.

What's exciting about that is since our thoughts, feelings, words, and actions create the world around us, we have the power to create a world of peace, harmony, and abundance.

I've chosen to share just a few of those laws to help you understand how that is all possible.

## The Law of Abundance

The Law of Abundance states that we live in an abundant universe. There is plenty of everything, including love, money, and all the necessities for everyone.

The key to having abundance is alignment with the conditions for manifesting it.

You likely grew up hearing things like "there are starving children in Africa, so you need to eat every last bite of food that is on your plate." Or "money doesn't grow on trees."

The truth is, there is abundance in the world. It is all around you. It's about what you are choosing to focus on. We don't have any issues with scarcity in the world, even when it comes to those starving children. The planet produces enough food. Hunger is not a problem caused by nature. Hunger is caused by lack of efficiency and politics.

I am illustrating how it does not serve any of us well to confuse issues like hunger, not to be ignored, with scarcity.

The Abundance Mindset

How you view the world can affect the opportunities you see, your beliefs, and ultimately your results. You can choose to see the world as a place of abundance or a place of scarcity.

An abundance mindset is hopeful, positive, and expects the best. It is also more altruistic, since you believe you'll receive what you need. It frees you up to do more for others.

A scarcity mindset, on the other hand, leads to negativity and selfishness. You feel the need to look out for yourself, even at the expense of others.

| Abundance Mindset | Scarcity Mindset |
| --- | --- |
| There is plenty to go around. Everyone can win. | There is a limited supply of everything, and someone else must lose for you to win. |
| Life is easier. You believe anything is possible. Expect the best and things eventually go your way. | Life is difficult. Success is hard. You expect the worst and that's how it turns out. |

| | |
|---|---|
| Opportunities are easier to spot. | Opportunities are scarce, and you struggle to find them. |
| You take more risks. The bigger the risk, the bigger the reward. | You play it safe. You're afraid to lose. |
| You are more relaxed. You enjoy life because all your needs are met. | You live in fear and pessimism. You must fight the world to get what you want and need. |

Which view do you normally see the world through? Abundance or scarcity?

One way to begin feeling the abundance, which may seem counter intuitive, is by giving more. Whatever resource you feel you lack, give that.

It feels good to give and it tricks you into believing you have plenty, which changes your energy and puts you into the flow of abundance.

## How to Move from Scarcity to Abundance

1. Focus on what you already have. When you see that you already have enough, you feel abundant and are likely to attract more to you.

2. Avoid people that complain a lot. Complainers have a scarcity mindset. You're more susceptible to others' mindsets than you think. Spend time with positive people who have the mindset you want.

3. Visualize an abundant future. Instead of worrying about what you don't have, allow yourself to dream about what you want to achieve in the future.

4. Keep a positive journal. List the things in your life you feel grateful for. Be sure to mention all the people in your life. You probably have a home, a job, a car, family, friends, and so on. That's a good place to start.

5. Be generous. Demonstrate to yourself there is enough for everyone by sharing what you have, including time. The more you share, the more others want to reciprocate.

An abundance mindset won't magically put you into a Mercedes or add a few zeros to your bank account overnight. However, an abundance mindset will allow you to move forward with confidence as you take the necessary steps to make positive changes in your life.

# 17.Learn to See The Bright Side of Everything

Four Habits to Develop Which Lead to Positive Thinking

1. Pray

Yes, you might find this to be a cliché, but it's true. When you pray, you are calm, and your mind is peaceful; it will seem as if all your worries are far away. Some of you may say, "But Andrian, I can't pray, I don't know how." Yes, you can. Praying is just like talking to a friend, and God is your friend.

You may not have something simply because you haven't asked for it yet. So ask God. He is always there for you, always listening to you. Ask, and you will notice your mind becoming more positive.

2. Read Great Books

Will Smith said there are two keys to success: running and reading. (We're going to focus more on the reading side.) He also said there are billions of people who have already gone through what you're going through right now. Whatever it is, the answer to your problem has probably already been written in a book, an article, a blog or somewhere else on the Internet. He's right. You can find a solution to any problem simply by "Googling" it!

Take note: When I refer to "great books" I'm not talking about the novel-type of entertainment books. The great books I am talking about are those books that enhance you, nurture you, and help you become a better person. I'm talking about self-improvement books, success books, biographies of successful people, motivational books, and many other great books.

If you read a great book for just 20 minutes a day, you will accumulate 120 hours of learning in a year.

As Jim Rohn said, "Success is something you attract by the person you become." So if you want to have more, you must become more.

Also, reading a book changes the way you think. You'll notice, as you read positive books, that your thinking will be more positive, too. That's one of the secrets of successful people.

3. Listen to Faith-Building / Motivational Messages

Every morning, I love to listen to faith-building messages. It really affects my mind and causes me to become more calm, peaceful, and positive. When we hear something repeatedly, we begin to believe it.

Personally, I listen to Terri Savelle Foy's YouTube podcasts. I stumbled upon her about 3 months ago. I really like listening to her because of her sound advice in different areas of life such as goal-setting, achieving your dreams, fulfilling your purpose, breaking soul ties, finances and faith, and more. You'll definitely learn a lot from her. I also love to listen to the "Top 10 Success Rules of Highly Successful People" on the YouTube channel of Evan Carmichael. He features the Top 10 rules of well-known people such as Bill Gates, Warren Buffet, Mark Zuckerberg and others.

Maybe you've heard the phrase, "Automobile University." Many successful people grow their minds by listening to great audios during their travel time to and from work every day. They use the time spent in their automobile to put positive, faith-building, motivational, inspirational thoughts into their minds.

So, make sure you have something to listen to during your commute that can inspire you, motivate you, encourage you, and build your faith. You'll notice your mind becoming more positive day by day.

4. Say Positive Words / Affirmations

One of the most effective ways to train your mind to stay in a state of positive thinking is to always speak positive words, or affirmations, to yourself. Your words are very powerful, so always use them for good.

Yes, that one alone will drastically change your life if you say it more often.

Those are just some of the affirmations I use in my life. You can incorporate these, and more, into your life.

Once again, friend, use your words to empower, to motivate, to inspire, and to bless yourself and others. Inject positive words into every conversation. Stay positive – think positive.

Those are the things we can do to develop the habit of positive thinking. I'm sure, if you start doing them, within a month you will become a more peaceful, calm, happy, and positive person.

Again, as a recap, here are the four habits we can develop which lead to positive thinking:

1. Pray
2. Read Great Books
3. Listen to Faith-Building / Motivational Messages
4. Say Positive Words / Affirmations

I have incorporated these habits into my life, and my mindset is now tuned into a more positive vibration. You will notice you are happier the moment you begin practicing these four amazing habits. So remember: Think positively at all times. By changing our thinking, we change our lives.

## 7 Ways to Gain Confidence and Increase Self-Esteem

What is one of the most common problems in the world today? Low self-esteem (or low confidence).

Yes, this one aspect of life has a major impact on achieving success and attaining our goals. But why do you think most people have low self-esteem? And have you ever wondered, "How do I gain confidence and self-esteem?"

Maybe it was in the past, or maybe you are still experiencing it – that feeling of Why is this happening to me? – that feeling of anxiety, low self-esteem, or low confidence in yourself.

Why? Well, I don't have the specific answer for the question 'why' but I do have an answer to that specific question 'how'.

Let's Tackle 7 Ways to Gain Confidence and Self-Esteem:

1. Take Action

Have you ever noticed when you want to do something which you think is difficult, it can be very hard to get started? You procrastinate because your mind thinks of so many other things you need to do first. At the same time, the longer you put it off, the more your confidence shrinks and your self-esteem lowers. Why?

Because your subconscious mind is continually telling you that you have this big, difficult task to do, and until you complete it, you feel an emptiness within which lowers your energy.

Did you know that once you do those bigger tasks, and complete them, you will feel lighter? The weight will be lifted from your shoulders, and you will be able to say, "Wow, I'm very proud of myself! I have completed it." "Yes! Success!" "Completed and done – let's celebrate!"

That sense of completeness, of relief, will definitely increase your confidence and self-esteem.

So, if you're struggling to get that big task done, do something about it. Take action; break it up into little pieces. Do it bite by bite, one thing at a time. Focus on just one small task before moving on to the next one. Feel the satisfaction of each accomplishment you've made, and be proud of yourself.

Little by little, your confidence will grow, and your self-esteem will go up.

The most difficult part of accomplishing anything is the beginning. But once you start, you will realize you're in the flow and ready to encounter anything that comes your way. You are now unstoppable.

So, friend, always take action immediately when you need to do a task. You will see your confidence and self-esteem increase as you take more and more action.

2. Groom Yourself; Dress Nicely

When you look at yourself in the mirror, do you like what you see? Do you feel your hairstyle is appropriate, and that you look nice?

Have you ever noticed when you get dressed up that your attitude immediately changes? That your confidence is lifted a bit higher? That your self-esteem is rising?

Studies have shown that what you wear affects your confidence.

Therefore, to feel more confident and boost your self-esteem, get into the habit of dressing nicely. Even at home, try to dress nicely: style your hair, wear clothes that make you feel good about yourself, splash on some cologne/perfume that you like, smile, hold your head up high, pull your shoulders back, and feel handsome/beautiful.

Every day, friend, groom yourself and dress nicely. You will notice your confidence growing and your self-esteem increasing every single day.

3. Be with Positive People

Have you ever been in a conversation where all of the topics seem to drain your energy because they are mostly negative? How do you feel after having conversations such as these with your friends? Are these conversations nurturing? Do they lift you, or anyone else, up?

The answer is obviously no; they drain your energy. If you want to gain confidence and self-esteem, you need to be around positive people. You must consciously choose to be with people who nurture you, encourage you, and believe in you.

You can join a local Christian church where people are encouraging, accommodating, and supportive of you. A solid Christian church will show you love, hope, and encouragement. The members will not judge you but love you for who you are.

Another option is to join a community online. These communities are often very accommodating, helpful, and friendly.

I've been in one particular online community for about a month now. In this community, I'm not only learning a lot about online business, but I'm also getting lots of useful training and encountering wonderful people every day; people who are there to help me, support me with my endeavors and encourage me as we travel this journey together.

They are people who are willing to help, true people who are always there to support you. If you find yourself alone, try joining an online community. There you will not only learn a lot, but you will also meet some wonderful people along the way who will guide you, help you, nurture you, and encourage you every single day.

So, friend, be with positive people. Be part of a community and gain more confidence and self-esteem along the way.

4. Speak Up

Have you ever been at a conference or seminar, where the speaker finishes speaking and asks the audience if there are any questions, and everyone looks down to avoid being called on? Or, maybe you've been in a conversation with a group of people, and everybody is talking and sharing while you're only listening and not sharing or speaking up?

While there is nothing wrong with being quiet, always remember it is the people who ask for things who receive them. It's the people who speak up. It's the people who make their voices heard who make a difference. It's the people who speak up who usually act on their ideas. They aren't necessarily the most self-confident or well-educated people, but they're the brave people. They're the ones who overcame their shyness and fears and spoke anyway – those who felt the fear and acted anyway.

When you're afraid of speaking up, always remember this: You are a human being like everyone else. Everyone has their own worries, concerns, and fears. You are not that much different from anyone else. So, be human; be yourself. Never be afraid of people, or what they say about you.

Life is short, and you only have one life to live. Speak up – always – this is one of the most important things you can do to improve your confidence and self-esteem.

Whenever you're at a conference or seminar, be the first to speak up and ask a question. Whenever you're in a group, and you're brainstorming, be the first to suggest an idea. Whenever you meet someone you know, be the first to start the conversation. Whenever you feel you need to talk to a stranger, be the first to act.

Friend, there's power – and confidence – in being the first to speak. Afterward, you can relax and bask in the knowledge that you took that first step and spoke up.

Always speak up. Remember that you are important. Believe in yourself. You are wonderfully created by our Almighty God, so never be afraid to speak up.

Let your voice be heard. Hold your head high. Let your confidence and self-esteem be apparent to everyone. Speak up!

5. Start Speaking Positive Words to Yourself

Read this out loud: "I love you."

Did you hear that? Keep reading.

"I'm so proud of you."

"I believe in you."

"You're awesome."

"You're great."

"You're incredible."

"You're amazing."

Did you hear your voice saying those words? Those words must come from you, from inside you.

If you're not hearing them, then start saying them – now!

Always say positive things about and to yourself. You might not realize it, but you are always talking to yourself. Every minute, every second, every moment. Conversations are always happening in your head. Your mind is always talking, so be aware of what you say to yourself.

Always say something positive about yourself. Things like:

"You are beautiful/handsome."

"You can do it."

"You are kind and generous."

"You are a champion."

"You are special and unique."

"You are magnificent."

"You are happy, healthy, and prosperous."

"You are an amazing child of God."

"You are wonderful."

Start repeating positive things about yourself – every day, every hour, every minute, and every second.

Words are powerful. Utilize the power of your words; speak positively. Speak life!

6. Prepare and Plan

How else can you gain confidence and self-esteem? Through preparation and planning.

Preparation is key to building your confidence and self-esteem.

Have you ever been at a job interview and found yourself speechless halfway through because you didn't know what to say? Or have you ever taken an exam when you didn't have time to review the material? Or maybe you've had to give a report and found yourself stuttering through it because you didn't have time to prepare.

Planning is another key to building your confidence and self-esteem.

Yes, preparation and planning ahead of time are absolutely essential if you want to gain confidence and self-esteem; they can give you the gift of time. A little time spent preparing and planning today can give us free time tomorrow.

Some of you may be asking, "But Andrian, how can I prepare and plan?"

To prepare and plan, be strategic. First, list all the things you need to accomplish. Schedule them – hour by hour.

Do this for the whole day, including meal and break times. For example:

5:30-6:00 AM – Daily devotions (Bible reading and prayer)

6:00-6:45 AM – Breakfast, prep for day (bathing, getting dressed, etc.)

6:45-7:30 AM – Daily commute to work (listen to faith-building podcasts)

Keep going like this until your bedtime – and schedule your bedtime, too. Scheduling makes you more likely to do things because it lets your brain know there is a time to do each task.

Also, you will notice your tasks for the day are easier to remember and follow once you've written them down. It doesn't take long – you can make a schedule for your whole day in about 5 minutes.

You want to control your life? Then, you need to control your time. Your life is your time. If you want to plan your life, plan your time.

Friend, when you are prepared and have plans, then you will gain more confidence and self-esteem. At the same time, you will have more peace within, and you'll feel you are really in control of your life.

# 18.Gratitude Affirmations

Gratitude is the foundation for living in a state of abundance and without it, you won't find true fulfilment as your mind never appreciates the abundance you already have. Think about it, you live better than a king did just a couple of centuries ago. One could argue that you even life better than a king did only a couple of decades ago since you have such useful technology at your disposal. I among many other people also believe that gratitude will attract more good things into one's life, including wealth. So, when you go through these affirmations, aim to feel gratitude and express them as if you're the wealthiest person in the world. Speak them with confidence and use your body in a way that will create emotion. Remember that motion creates emotion so by using your body in a confident way, you'll benefit the most from these affirmations.

- I am grateful for living in the 21th century.
- I am so thankful for all the money that I have.
- I feel appreciation for the things money allows me to buy.
- I love life and I'm so grateful to be a part of it.
- I know that life is a gift.
- While I inhale, I take full pleasure of the air that energizes my body and mind.
- I am so grateful for the opportunities life has given me.
- I'm so grateful for the opportunities life is continuing to give me.

- I feel gratitude towards people for I know that they can help me achieve my dreams.
- I am so grateful for who I am since I know that I can create magnificent things.
- I am grateful for being in control.
- I feel grateful for the people in my life.
- I am grateful for the opportunities to come.
- I was given the gift of life and the chance to make whatever I want of it, and for that I am grateful.
- I am grateful for all the resources that I have and those that are to come.
- I am grateful for my resourcefulness and my ability to find solutions.
- I see the good in events and people.
- I know that the chances of me being born were very low and I am so grateful for beating the odds.
- Gratitude is my antidote to fear and anger. I am now in control of my emotions.
- I am so grateful for my ability to produce.
- Every day, I am living life to the fullest as a thanks to God for giving me the gift of life.
- I am so grateful for my prosperous future.
- I am grateful for my health, wealth, love and happiness.
- An abundance of money is flowing to me right now and for that I am grateful.

- I am so grateful that people treat me with respect and care for my well-being.
- I am so grateful for having all my needs meet.
- I give thanks to the Universe for allowing me to live my dreams.
- I am the master of my life and for that, I am grateful.
- I am so grateful for being able to use the wonderful things that others have created.
- I am grateful for all the money ideas that come to me.
- I know that one only needs to be right one time to become financially prosperous and I am grateful that it's my turn now.
- I am grateful for I know that successful people want to help me, be it via books, videos or in person.
- I am grateful for the abundance of choices I've been given.
- I know that freedom is uncertain for some people in other parts of the world, that's why I appreciate that I've been born here.
- I am grateful for money.
- I am free to live life on my own terms, and for that I am grateful.
- I am grateful for the plenty of opportunities to create an abundance of money.
- I know that my mind can create incredible things and for that, I am grateful.
- I am so grateful for having multiple sources of income.
- I am so grateful that money comes to me in avalanches of abundance from unexpected sources on a continuous basis.

- I love all the events money can allow me to experience.
- I am grateful for my incredible ability to solve problems and bring immense value to the market place.
- I am grateful for my commitment to live in abundance.
- I know that I can feel the feeling of abundance whenever I want, and for that I am so grateful.
- I hereby give thanks to the Universe for all the prosperity I experience.
- Money flows effortlessly to me and for that, I am grateful.
- Gratitude is a gift of life and I experience it daily.
- Abundance is a natural state for me and I love it.
- I live better than hundreds of kings before me and for that, I am grateful.
- I am so grateful that money flows with ease into my bank account.
- Every day, and in every way, I'm experiencing more and more joy in my life.
- Happiness is my natural state.
- I deserve to be happy.
- By being happy, I help others to become happy.
- I am so grateful for the joyful feeling that follows me everywhere.
- I spread happiness to others and absorb happiness from others.

- I am so happy and grateful now that my outlook on life is positive.
- Being happy is easy for me.
- I am grateful for every moment of every day for I know it shall never return.
- My future is bright, and I am so thankful for it.
- I think uplifting thoughts.
- Life is easy for me.
- I am grateful for the air I'm breathing, the water I got access to and the food in my fridge.
- I always have what I need and for that, I'm grateful.
- I start everyday in a state of happiness and joy.
- I am a joyful giver and a happy receiver of good things in my life.
- I am meant to be here in this world and fulfil a purpose.
- The world will be a better and happier place because I was here.
- I am an unstoppable force for good.
- I trust myself, my inner wisdom knows the truth.
- I forgive myself and others for all the mistakes made.
- I breathe in happiness with every breath I take.
- This day brings me happiness.
- I wake up feeling grateful for life.
- Today is my day to shine light on the world.

- Everything always works out for the best for me.
- I trust the Universe to guide me to my true calling in life.
- I am so happy and grateful now that I get to live my dream.
- I am always improving and learning new things.
- I am present and feel joy in this moment.
- I can transform any negative into a positive.
- I am a positive person with incredible gifts to give to the world.
- I am the creator of my day, my weeks, my months and my years.
- I decide to make my life a masterpiece worth remembering.
- I feel alive and the world around me feels fresh and new.
- I breathe deeply and connect with my inner being.
- Thank you, thank you, thank you.
- Life is wonderful, and I love living.
- There are endless opportunities to experience joy and happiness every day.
- I transform obstacles into opportunities.
- I am eternally grateful for the abundance in my life.
- I make a conscious decision to be happy.
- My life is overflowing with happiness and joy.
- I am so grateful that I get to live another day.
- The world is a beautiful place.

- I deserve whatever great comes my way today.
- I am a great receiver of wonderful things and experiences.
- I am a magnet that always attract positive things and events.
- I believe in myself.
- I am a confident person with a positive mindset.
- I always have more than enough to be happy.
- I live an uplifting life and I always attract positive things into it.
- Time is my most valuable asset; I therefore spend it in the best way possible.
- I always hold the power to decide what I wish to do with my life.
- I love life and life loves me.
- The Universe is guiding me towards my higher purpose in life.
- I am in full control of my thoughts and emotions.
- I allow myself to have fun and enjoy life.
- I am at peace with a tremendous amount of happiness and joy.
- I trust that what's happening is happening for the greater good.
- I create a vision for my life and a plan to achieve it.
- I trust my ability to find solutions.
- The Universe is always looking out for me.
- Today, I am feeling confident and strong.
- This day is another well written page in my life's book.

- I only compare myself to my highest self.
- I am grounded and secure in my being.
- I surround myself with positive people who want the best for me.
- I am a patient, calm and loving individual who is on the right path in life.
- I live right here and now and accept the present moment.
- I am grateful and joyful to live another day in this beautiful world.
- I realize that I hold a tremendous amount of knowledge that can be used for good.
- My experiences are unique to me and there's personal power in that.
- I guide and help other gracious people with my experience and wisdom.
- My uniqueness makes me uniquely successful.
- I take one step at the time and always trust that I will reach my destination.
- I am so happy and grateful for all the blessings in my life.
- My being is overflowing with creative energy.
- I am in perfect harmony with life.
- I am at peace with who I am.
- I am at peace with other people.
- It's easy for me to live in abundance and prosperity.

- I find it easy to be confident.
- I greet the day with ease.
- I praise people when they do something good that I honestly appreciate.
- I praise and reward myself when I do something good.
- I encourage others and always see the full potential of what they can be.
- Every day, and in every way, I'm getting more and more confident.
- I now realize the preciousness of life.
- I attract happy and kind people into my life.
- I am so grateful for the kindness of others.
- I am so grateful for my strengths.
- I make the right decisions with ease.
- I am so happy and grateful now that I get to experience life with a positive mindset.
- I am a master at creating long-lasting habits that have a positive impact on my life.
- I radiate happiness, joy, confidence and graciousness.
- Being and staying positive is easy for me.
- I am open to the goodness of the Universe.
- All my actions lead me to happiness and abundance.
- I am so grateful for having all I need to be happy right now.

# 19.Abundance Affirmations

To live a life of true abundance, we first must make a conscious decision to live in a beautiful state no matter what. Life does not happen to us, it happens for us and with that knowledge in mind, we can trust that the Universe is taking care of us and guiding us to the person we want to be as well as our desired place. So trust the process and choose to relax by breathing deeply whenever challenges arise. They are put in place to make you who God has intended you to be.

- Gods wealth is circulating in my life.
- I hereby chose to live in a beautiful state.
- The Universe has my best interest at heart.
- I experience avalanches of abundance and all my needs are met instantaneously.
- Abundance is something we tune in to.
- I choose to live in abundance in every moment of everyday for the rest of my life.
- I know that I am being guided to my true self.
- I live in financial abundance.
- I know that my needs are always met and that answers are given to me.
- Everyday in every way, I am becoming more and more abundant.

- The Universe takes good care of me as I always have what I need.
- My life is full of all the material things I need.
- My life is filled with joy and love.
- Money flows to me in abundance.
- I have everything in abundance.
- Prosperity overflows in my life.
- My thoughts are always about prosperity and abundance.
- My actions lead to prosperity and abundance.
- I hereby focus on prosperity and abundance and thereby attract it into my life.
- Abundance and prosperity is within me as well as around me.
- I hereby allow all great things to come into my life.
- I enjoy the good things that flows into my life.
- I create prosperity easily and effortlessly.
- I feel passionate about prosperity and thus it comes to me naturally.
- I love abundance and I naturally attract it.
- The whole Universe is conspiring to make me abundant and prosperous.
- I let go of any resistance to abundance and prosperity and it comes to me naturally.
- I am grateful for the prosperity and abundance in my life.

- I am open and receptive to all the prosperity life is now willing to give me.
- I am surrounded by prosperity.
- I deserve to be wealthy.
- My visions are becoming a reality.
- Thank you Universe for all that you've given me.
- I am a money magnet.
- Prosperity is naturally drawn to me.
- I am always using abundance thinking.
- I am worthy of becoming financially prosperous.
- I am one with the energy of abundance.
- I use money to better my life as well as the lives of others.
- I am the master of money
- Money is my worker.
- I can handle large sums of money.
- I enjoy having an abundance of money.
- I am at peace with large sums of money flowing to me.
- Money leads to opportunities and experiences.
- An abundance of money creates positive impact in my life.
- It's my birthright to live in a state of abundance.
- The Universe is guiding me to more prosperity right now.

- Money is coming to me in large quantities and I am ready for it.
- People want me to live in abundance and I know I deserve it.
- Wealth creates a positive, fulfilling, and rewarding impact on my life.
- I realize that money is important for leading a wonderful life.
- The Universe is a constant provider of money and wealth for me, and I have more than enough wealth to meet all my needs.
- My actions and activities make more money for me, and I am constantly supplied with money.
- My bank balance increases each day, and I always have more than enough money and wealth for myself.
- Wealth and I are buddies and we'll always be together.
- Each day I attract and save more and more money.
- Money is an integral aspect of my life and has never gone away from me.
- I am free of debt, as money, wealth, and abundance are forever flowing in my life.
- My money consciousness is forever increasing and has kept me surrounded by wealth, money, and abundance.
- I have a highly positive wealth and money mindset.
- I am highly focused on becoming wealthy, rich, and prosperous.
- Attracting wealth, money, and abundance is easy.
- My bank account value is growing by the day.
- Money is wonderful energy.

- My wealth and income automatically rise higher and higher.
- I let myself enjoy each moment of my day.
- I always chase my bliss.
- I always look for ways to attract more joy and laughter into my life.
- I am complete within myself.
- I am everything I choose to be.
- I am healthy, happy, joyful, and strong.
- Everything I need to be is within me.
- I completely believe in myself and everything that I have to give the world.
- I am bold, courageous, and brave.
- I am free to create the life of my dreams and desires.
- I am present, mindful, and aware.
- The possibilities that life presents me with are infinite.
- I am open to receiving.
- I float happily and in a content manner within my world.
- I deserve to be in a serene, calm, and peaceful state.
- I choose to live a happy, balanced, and peaceful life.
- I create a place of peace, tranquility and harmony for myself and others.
- I find happiness, joy, and pleasure in the tiniest of things.

- I can tap into my spring of internal happiness anytime I desire and let out a flow of joy, pleasure, happiness, and well-being.
- I look at and observe the world with a smile, because I can't help but sense the joy around me.
- I have great fun with even the most mundane of endeavors.
- I have a wonderful sense of humor and love to share laughter and joy with others.
- My heart is overflowing with a feeling of happiness and joy.
- I rest in complete bliss and happiness each time I go to sleep, knowing only too well that everything is fine in my Universe.
- Happiness is my right. I wholeheartedly embrace happiness as my state of being.
- I am the most content and happiest person on this planet.
- I am glad that all happiness originates from within me and I live every moment to the fullest.
- I wake up every day with a joyful smile on my face and a sense of gratitude in my heart for all the wonderful moments that await me during the day.

# 16.Affirmations About Attracting Money

Money tends to come to those who have a prosperity mindset. The gratitude and abundance affirmations that we've gone through have lifted up your invisible money magnet so you can start attracting an abundance of wealth into your life. You've probably heard at least one of these ridiculous statements before. Let's break each of these wacky sayings down, shall we?

Nr 1: Money is the root of all evil. Money is simply a means of exchange. Do you prefer we go back to barter? Finding someone who will want to change your apple for a pen will be both frustrating and time consuming. Money is neither good or bad. Yes indeed, you can do both good and bad things with money but stating that money itself is evil is just ludicrous. Think about all the good things people have done with money, all the lives they have saved. Think about all the people with money who have created companies in which people can work and earn a living. Think about all the good things you can do with money and all the lives you can better. If you think this limiting belief is holding you back from living in financial abundance, consider using the following affirmation: Money is neutral and a resource to do good in my life.

Nr 2: Money can't buy happiness. As we've already the mentioned before, there are studies showing that money can increase one's happiness up to a certain point and perhaps even beyond. Even if the statement "money can't buy happiness" was true (which it's not), money can buy time. And more time, can surely make one happier. For example, if you have a lot of money, you can hire other people to do chores that you don't particularly enjoy doing. Also think about all the experiences that money can buy. Whenever we are focused on the negative, we need to stop and ask ourselves; "what are the opportunities?" If you want an affirmation that will absolutely turn this limiting belief into the small ball of dust it really is, consider the following one:

I love money as it can buy me both experiences and time with my loved ones.

Nr 3: Money is not everything. Of course it's not everything Dum-Dum, but you need it don't you? Or how do you get food on the table and a roof over your head? Let's follow the advice, "don't argue with a foolish argument", regarding this one and just move on to the next one, shall we?

Nr 4: People can make a lot of money, but they do it at the expense of their family. Some individuals may prioritize work over spending time with their family. However, this does not make the statement an absolute truth. People seldom get rich by hard work alone. People acquire great wealth by doing the right things. Such things include making their money work for them by making smart investments or leveraging other people's time and money. To crush this limiting belief, start searching for people who are making a lot of money who work less than the average worker. I'm sure you will come across a lot of people who have found a way to use leverage to make a lot of money, perhaps even in an automated way. Also, consider the fact that the average person in America is watching around 5 hours of television per day. Surely there doesn't seem to be a shortage of time to spend with loved ones if one prioritizes differently? Here's an affirmation to let you overcome this limiting belief: With more money, I can choose to spend more time with my family if I want to.

Nr 5: It's selfish to have a lot of money. As mentioned before, money is simply a means of exchange. In other words, you change your money for something you want, or vise versa. This means that you must have provided something of perceived value to someone else to receive that money. Again, providing value doesn't have to be linked with your time. Investors can for example provide value by letting other people provide value with the help of their money. Either way, acquiring money is neither a selfish or unselfish act, it's simply an exchange of value. If you struggle with this limiting belief, consider replacing it by using the following affirmations: The money I've earned reflects the value I've created for others. Hopefully this list, has helped you tackle the most disturbing false beliefs about money. If you think you have more, don't worry, the 50 money affirmations soon to come will surely help you overcome most of the silly associations that people tend to drop senselessly in to our mind as we get older. As Jim Rohn said, we must stay guard at the door of our mind every day! Now, as you may have heard before; you can give a man a fish to feed him for a day or you can teach him how to fish so he can feed himself for a lifetime. I'll aim to do both; so here's two noteworthy ideas for you to consider when overcoming any limiting beliefs, be it regarding money, love, health or happiness. First, ask yourself this one simple question: Is this belief an absolute truth for me as an individual or can I find people or circumstances that proves that the opposite can also be true? Secondly, as you might have already noted, I've used rather harsh adjectives to describe some of these limiting beliefs. The reason for this is because I want to break a pattern and the easiest way to do that is by strong emotion or doing something unexpected. You can also add a voice to the limiting belief that is impossible for you to take seriously (for example, a voice from a South Park character). Imagine this voice combined with a face you can't take seriously and then visualize how this face is blowing up as a balloon and becoming smaller and smaller as it's flying away to some distant corner. You can also write down the limiting belief, then scrunch the paper and throw it in a garbage can. Personally, I like the voice method the best, but you choose whichever method or methods that works best for you.

Are you ready to start with the affirmations? Okay, here we go!

- I'm filled with joy and gratitude and I love that more and more money is flowing to me continuously.
- Money is flowing to me in avalanches of abundance from unexpected sources.
- Money is coming to me faster and faster.
- I deserve prosperity and to have an abundance of money in my bank account.
- All my dreams, goals and desires are met instantaneously.
- The Universe is on my side and it is guiding me towards wealth.
- The Universe is guiding wealth towards me.
- I love money and all that it can buy.
- I feel grateful that I increase my net worth substantially every year.
- Money flows to me with ease.
- Ideas to make more money is coming to me often.
- I feel good about money.
- I can do good things with money.
- I am worthy of prosperity and having an abundance of money.
- I release all my negative beliefs about money and allow for financial abundance to enter.
- Money is always close to me.
- Opportunities to make more money come to me effortlessly.

- I give value and money loves me for it.
- I attract money with ease and I now have more wealth than I ever dreamed possible.
- I am wealthy, and I feel incredibly good about it.
- I have a great relationship with money.
- I am gracious for all the money that I have.
- Every day and in every way, I am attracting more money into my life.
- Being wealthy feels fantastic.
- I attract money effortlessly.
- I now allow for money to flow freely into my life.
- I am a money magnet and money will always be attracted to me.
- I am now relaxing into greater prosperity.
- I release all opposition to money.
- I deserve to have a lot of money in my bank account.
- Ideas of making money is freely entering my life.
- Abundance is all around me and I feel so gracious about it.
- Being wealthy is my natural state.
- The Universe is helping me to attract money into my life right now.
- I am prosperous, and I appreciate all the good things in my life.
- I am affluent.

- It feels phenomenal to have a lot of money in my bank account.
- I love money and money loves me.
- It's very easy for me to make more money.
- I am a natural born money maker.
- I am willing and ready to receive more money now.
- My income increases substantially each year.
- I happily receive money with ease.
- The Universe keeps giving me more and more money.
- Attracting money is easy for me.
- Money is good and with it I can help other people better their life.
- Financial success is my birth right.
- An avalanche of money is transporting itself to me.
- I feel good about receiving large quantities of money.
- Thank you Universe for allowing me to live in prosperity.
- I'm so grateful for living in prosperity.
- Every day, in every way, I'm attracting more and more money into my life.
- I live in abundance now.
- Money comes to me with ease.
- I see many opportunities for creating wealth.
- I give and receive with ease.

- I feel gratitude for all the money that I have.
- I'm a great giver; I'm also an exceptional receiver.
- By being wealthy and having a lot of money, I can make the world a better place.
- It feels fantastic to have a lot of money.
- The universe responds to my prosperity mindset by giving me more opportunities to make money with ease.
- I visualize being wealthy every day and I send out good vibrations about money.
- I'm a money magnet that attracts money from all types of places.
- I am abundant every day, in every way.
- I'm gracious for all the prosperity I receive.
- I pay myself first and my money multiplies.
- An avalanche of money is now entering my life.
- Making money is easy for me.
- I constantly find and come up with new ways to make more money with ease.
- Money is one important part of my life and I give it the time and attention it deserves.
- Money allows me to help more people.
- Money allows me to spend more time with my loved ones.
- Money allows me to have more wonderful experiences.
- Having more money is a good thing for me.

- I love money and all the wonderful things it can do.
- I love the freedom that money gives me.
- I deserve to be wealthy and to live in abundance.
- I attract money from all kinds of unexpected sources.
- I continuously have a big surplus of money at the end of every month.
- I am attracted to money and money is attracted to me.
- I continuously learn from other people who live in financial abundance be it via books, videos, audio or in person.
- My actions create a lot of value for others.
- I am a person of great value.
- I make my money work for me.
- My money brings me more money.
- I am a great money manager.
- I see more and more great opportunities for creating wealth.
- I am a multi-millionaire.
- I am so grateful for ability to make a lot of money.
- I am at one with a tremendous amount of money in my bank account.
- My financial reality is in my control alone.
- Money is my servant.
- I have everything I need to create financial abundance.

- There is enough money to create prosperity.
- Being rich is easy.
- I always have access to a lot of money.
- I am worthy of being affluent.
- I enjoy making money.
- I enjoy having multiple streams of passive income.
- I trust that the Universe always meets my needs.
- Wealth is showering and pouring into my life.
- The Universe's riches are drawn to me easily and effortlessly.
- I openly accept wealth, prosperity, and abundance now.
- I am grateful for the overflowing, unrestrained, and limitless source of wealth.
- Everything I turn my hand to returns riches and abundance.
- I am a money magnet. Money is always attracted to me.
- My life is completely filled with powerful and positive abundance.
- All my needs are more than met.
- I am prosperous and money gushes to me from multiple sources.
- I am the fortunate receiver of wealth flowing from several revenue streams.
- I give and receive graciously and I am a constantly flowing stream of wealth.

- I graciously accept all the happiness, abundance, and wealth the Universe showers me with each day.
- Income flows to me in unexpected ways.
- I love money and money loves me.
- All the money and wealth I want is flowing to me right now.
- I am an overflowing treasure trove of abundance.
- I easily, smoothly, and effortlessly attract financial prosperity, wealth, and abundance into each aspect of my life.
- I always have more than enough money.
- Money keeps flowing to me from expected and unexpected sources.
- Money constantly circulates in my life freely and effortlessly.
- There is always surplus money flowing to me.
- I am financially free.
- Money comes flying to me from several directions.
- Money comes to me generously in perfect ways.
- There is an abundance of things to love in my life and the lives of everyone around me.
- I am perennially adding to income and wealth.
- Money flows through me, and I have more than enough wealth to meet all my needs and wishes.
- Money is flowing to me each day.
- Money is drawn to me easily, effortlessly, and frequently.

- I am a prosperity magnet. Prosperity and abundance is always drawn to me.
- I think abundance all the time.
- I am completely worthy of attracting wealth and money into my life.
- I deserve wealth, money and abundance.
- I am open and accepting to receive the wealth and abundance life has to offer me.
- I embrace and celebrate new ways of generating income.
- I draw, welcome, and invite unlimited sources of wealth, money, and income into my life.
- I use money to better my own and other people's lives.
- I am fully aligned with the energy of wealth and abundance.
- My actions and deeds lead to continuous prosperity.
- I attract money and wealth creation opportunities.
- My finances are improving beyond my imagination.
- Wealth is the root of comfort, joy, and security.
- Money, spirituality, and contentment can completely coexist in harmony.
- Money, love, and happiness can all be friends.
- Money works for me.
- I am the master of money, wealth, and abundance.
- I am capable of handling huge sums of money.

- I am completely at peace having a lot of money.
- I can handle success with dignity and grace.
- Wealth expands my life's experiences, passions, and opportunities.

# 20. Self Esteem Affirmations

- I am willing to accept mistakes. They are the stepping stones to success.
- I am always learning and growing.
- I will not compare myself to others.
- I focus on the things I can change.
- I deserve a good life. I toss away the ideas of suffering and misery.
- I love myself as I am.
- I am constantly growing and changing for the better.
- I am smart, competent, and able.
- I believe in myself, in my skills, and in my abilities.
- I am useful and make contributions to society and my own life.
- My decisions are sound and reasonable, and I stand by them.
- I have the capability to acquire all the knowledge I need to succeed.
- I am free to make my own decisions and choices.
- I am worthy of others' respect.
- I accept compliments easily and give them freely.
- I accept other people as they are, which in turn allows them to accept me as I am.

- I respect myself.
- I let go of the need to prove myself to others. I am my own self, and I love me as I am.
- I am full of courage. I am willing to act despite fear.
- I trust myself.
- I approach strangers with enthusiasm and boldness.
- I breathe in a manner that helps me to feel more confident. I inhale confidence and exhale timidity.
- I am confident of my future.
- I am a self-reliant, persistent, and creative person in everything I do.
- I make confidence my second nature.
- I am able to find the best solution to my problems.
- I remember that nothing is impossible.
- I am unique. I feel good. I love living life and being me.
- I have integrity.
- I accept myself fully.
- I am proud of myself.
- I allow my mind to fill up with nourishing and positive thoughts.
- I accept myself and find inner peace in doing so.
- I have the ability to overcome all challenges that life gives me.
- I am capable of rising up in the face of adversity.

- I make my own decisions and choices.
- I deserve to be happy and successful.
- I hold the power and potential to change myself for the better
- I can make my own choices and decisions.
- I am free to make my own choices and decisions.
- I can choose to live as I want while giving priority to my desires, goals, and dreams.
- I pick happiness each time I want, irrespective of the circumstances.
- I am open, adaptive, and flexible to change in each sphere of my life.
- I operate from a position of confidence, self-assuredness, and high self-esteem each day of my life.
- I always do my best.
- I am deserving of the love I receive.
- I like meeting strangers and approaching them with enthusiasm, interest and boldness.
- I am creative, perseverant and self-reliant in everything I do.
- I appreciate change and quickly adapt myself to new circumstances.
- I always observe the positive in others.
- I am one of a kind. I feel wonderful about being alive, being happy, and being me.
- Life is rewarding, fun, and enjoyable.

- There are a lot of awesome opportunities for me in all aspects of life.
- My life is full of opportunities everywhere.
- Challenges always bring out the best in me.
- I replace "must," "should," and "have to" with "choose," and notice the difference.
- I choose to be in a state of happiness right now. I enjoy my life.
- I appreciate all that is happening in my life now. I really love my life.
- I live in a place of joy.
- I am brave, courageous, and fearless.
- I am positive, optimistic, and always believe that things will turn out best.
- It is easy for me to make friends as I attract positive, compassionate and kind people into my life.
- I am a powerful creator because I make the life I desire.
- I am alright because I love and accept myself as I am.
- I completely trust myself, and I am a confident person.
- I am successful in my life right now.
- I am passionate, enthusiastic and inspiring.
- I have peace, serenity, calmness, and positivity.
- I am optimistic that everything will work out only for the best.

- I have unlimited resources, power, confidence, and positivity at my disposal.
- I am kind, loving, and compassionate, and care about others
- I am persistent, perseverant, and focused. I never quit.
- Self-confidence is my second skin. I am energetic, passionate and enthusiastic.
- I treat everyone with kindness, compassion, and respect.
- I inhale self-confidence and exhale doubts.
- I am flexible and adapt to change instantly.
- I possess endless reserves of integrity. I am reliable and do exactly what I say I will.
- I am smart and intelligent.
- I am competent and capable.
- I completely believe in myself.
- I recognize and identify all the good qualities I possess.
- I am fabulous, glorious, and awesome. There's no one else like me.
- I always see the best in everyone around me.
- I surround my life with people who bring out the best in me.
- I release negative thoughts and feelings I have about myself.
- I love the person I become each day.
- I am forever growing, nurturing, and developing.
- My opinions match who I truly am.

- I deserve all the happiness and success in the world.
- I possess the power to change myself.
- I am competent in making my own choices and decisions.
- I have complete freedom to choose to live the way I want, and give priority to my desires and wishes.

# 21.Self-Love Affirmations

- I am surrounded by love.
- I keep my heart open.
- I radiate love.
- I deserve to love and be loved in return.
- I always get what I give out into the world.
- I am able to see from my partner's point of view, so I am able to understand my partner perfectly.
- I am able to express my feelings openly.
- All of my relationships offer a positive and loving experience.
- I am happy to give and receive love every day.
- I am grateful for how loved I am, and how much people care about me.
- I have the power to give love endlessly.
- I welcome love with open arms.
- I allow my inner beauty to radiate outward.
- My relationships fulfill me.
- I am beautiful.
- I trust in the universe to find me my perfect match.
- I feel love. I see love. I am loved.

- I love myself and every aspect of my life.
- I look at everything with loving eyes, and I love everything I see.
- My partner loves me for who I am.
- I respect and admire my partner.
- I see the best in my partner.
- I share emotional intimacy with those I have a strong relationship with.
- My partner and I communicate openly.
- I am able to resolve conflicts with my loved ones in a peaceful and respectful manner.
- I am able to be myself in a romantic relationship.
- I support my partner and want the best for him/her.
- I deserve compassion, empathy, and love.
- I have a caring and warm heart.
- I am filled with love for who I am.
- My life is filled with love.
- Love flows through me in every situation.
- I find love wherever I go.
- I am able to receive love with open arms.
- I am supported by my family, friends, relationships, and I love it.
- I am willing to allow joy in my life.

- I show joy to all that I interact with.
- I choose joy. It is a possibility in each and every moment of my life.
- My day begins and ends with joy and gratitude for myself.
- My experiences in joy expand every day.
- I let myself feel appreciation and joy for the people who love me.
- I give myself permission to feel joy.
- I allow myself to be open to experiencing more joyous moments every day.
- My words, actions, and thoughts support my joyful living.
- I choose joy to be a part of my inner self.
- I am happy with all of my achievements.
- I make choices and decisions that nurture me and bring me joy.
- I greet every day with gratitude and joy.
- I am allowed to feel joy.
- I let myself concentrate on thoughts that make me happy.
- I give joy away to others so I can receive it in return.
- I understand that it is okay to feel joy when others do not.
- Experiencing life brings me great joy.
- One joyful experience opens up the door to many more joyful experiences.
- I allow my joy to empower me to new heights.

- I smile and feel joy at the world around me.
- Even the simple things in life allow me to feel joy.
- I feel joy in being alive.
- I am able to find joy in the simple things.
- I love to share my joy with others.
- I am able to find joy in every moment that happens.
- I welcome joy into my life.
- I am able to accept joy and peace in all aspects of my life.
- I let go of all anxiety, worry, fear, and doubt, and fill myself with peace, love, and joy.
- I create a home full of joy.
- I do my best every day, which fills me with joy.
- I share freely the joy I feel in my heart.
- I enjoy doing nice things for other people.
- My everyday responsibilities give my life balance and joy.
- I am able to make whatever I am doing enjoyable.
- I am filled with light, love, and peace
- I treat myself with kindness and respect
- I give myself permission to shine
- I honor the best parts of myself and share them with others
- I am proud of all that I have accomplished

- Today I give myself permission to be greater than my fears
- I am my own best friend and cheerleader
- I have many qualities, traits, and talents that make me unique
- I am a valuable human being
- I love myself just the way I am
- I love and forgive myself for any past mistakes
- I look in the mirror and I love what I see
- I recognize my many strengths
- I choose happiness each day, irrespective of my external circumstances.
- I can confidently speak my mind.
- I have respect for others, which makes others like and respect me in return.
- My thoughts, opinions, and actions are invaluable.
- I am confident that I can accomplish everything I want today and every day.
- I have something wonderful and special to offer the world.
- People love, admire, and respect me.
- I am an amazing person who feels great about myself and my wonderful life.

# 22. Relax Affirmations

The best way to include these affirmations in your life is to repeat them daily. They will help retrain your brain to think more positively rather than the negative ways that you might be thinking now.

In order to reiterate the importance of affirmations, including physical activity can help you to remember them even more. When you integrate a physical exercise with a mental thought, it helps make it more real. It will be easier to accept these affirmations in your life when an emphasis is put on truly believing them.

The first movement that you can do in order to remember these exercises is to physically hold an item. It can be something as small as a stone that you keep in your pocket, or you can pick out a special pillow or blanket that you choose to use with each affirmation.

As you are saying these affirmations, physically touch and hold these items. Let it remind you of reality. Stay focused and grounded on remembering the most important aspects of these affirmations.

Alternatively, try implementing new breathing exercises that we haven't tried yet. The method of breathing in through your nose and out through your mouth is important, but as we go further, there are other ways that you can include healthy breathing with these positive sleep affirmations.

One method is by breathing through alternate nostrils. Make a fist with your right hand with your thumb and pinky sticking out. Take your pinky and place it on your left nostril, closing it so that you can only breathe through one.

Now, breathing for five counts through that nostril.

Then, take your right thumb, and place it on your right nostril, closing that and releasing your pinky from the other nostril. Now, breathe out for five.

You will notice that doing this breathing exercise on its own is enough to help you be more relaxed. Now, when you pair it with the affirmation that we're about to read aloud, you will start to put more of an emphasis on creating thinking patterns around these affirmations.

An alternate method of breathing is to breathe in for three counts, say the affirmation, and then breathe out for three counts. You can do this on your own with the affirmations that are most important to your life.

It will be beneficial for you to have a journal that you keep affirmations in as well. Have one handy to write these affirmations down as they apply to your life. Writing about them will help you remember them and keep a note of the things that are most effective in your life.

When you are having a bad day, you can visit these affirmations. When you need a little confidence booster, or some motivation, use these affirmations.

We will now get into the reading of these. Remember to focus on your breathing as we take you through these, and if you are not planning on drifting off to sleep once they have finished, taking notes can help as well.

- I am dedicated to making healthy choices for my sleeping habits.
- The things that I do throughout my day will affect how I sleep; therefore, I am going to make sure to focus on making the best choices for all aspects of my health.
- I will do things that aren't always easy because it will be in the best interest of my health overall.
- When I am well-rested, everything else in my life become easier.

- I am more focused when I have slept an entire night, so I know that falling asleep is incredibly important to my health.
- Developing healthy habits is easy when I dedicate my time towards a better future.
- It feels good to take care of myself.
- I deserve a good night's sleep; therefore, I deserve everything else that will come along with this benefit.
- I am naturally supposed to get rest. It is not wrong for me to be tired and to choose to do healthy things for my sleep cycles.
- Dreams are normal, and I am focused on embracing them and avoiding nightmares.
- I choose to go to bed at a decent time at night because it is best for my health.
- Whatever is waiting for me tomorrow will still be there whether I get a full night's sleep or not, so it is best to ensure I am getting the proper amount of rest.
- I take care of my body because I know that it is the only one that I will ever have.
- I allow discipline in my life to guide me in the right direction to make the choices that are healthiest for my individual and specific lifestyle.
- I nourish my body and make sure I get the right amount of nutrients to keep me energized throughout the day.
- I am strong because I get the right amount of sleep.
- Getting the right kind of sleep is good for my mental health.

- I am happier when I am well-rested. I am in a better mood and can laugh more easily when I have had a good night's sleep.
- I am grateful for my opportunity to be healthier and to get better sleep.
- I am thankful that I have the ability to make the right choices for my health and overall well-being.
- Having habits is not a bad thing, I just need to make sure that my habits are healthy ones.
- I am less stressed out when I am able to get a better night's sleep.
- I am the best version of myself when I am healthy. I am healthiest when I am well-rested and focused on getting a better night's sleep.
- Everything else in my life will fall into place as I focus on getting the best night's sleep possible.
- I love myself, therefore I am going to put an emphasis on dedication to better sleeping habits so that I can feel better all the time.
- I am feeling relaxed.
- Relaxation is a feeling I can elicit, not a state that I have to be in depending on certain restrictions.
- I can feel the relaxation in my mind first and foremost.
- As I feel my body becoming relaxed, I can feel that serenity pass through the upper half of my body.
- All of the tension that I might have built throughout the day is now starting to fade away.
- I am focused on myself and centered within my body.

- I can tell that my muscles are becoming more and more relaxed.
- There is nothing that is concerning me at the moment.
- There will always be stressors in my life, but right now, I do not have to worry about any of those.
- As I focus on being calmer, it is easier for my mind to relax.
- I do not have to be afraid of what happened in the past.
- I cannot change the things that are already written in history.
- I don't need to be fearful of the future.
- I can make assumptions, but my predictions will not always be accurate.
- I can focus on the now, which is the most important thing to do.
- As I start to draw my attention to the present moment, I find it easier to relax.
- The more relaxed I am, the easier it will be for me to fall asleep.
- The faster I fall asleep, the more rest that I can get.
- I have no concern over what is going on around me. The only thing I am concerned with is being relaxed in the present moment.
- I exude relaxation and peace. Others will notice how quiet, calm, and collected I can be.
- I am balanced in my stress and pleasure aspects, meaning that I have less anxiety.
- I am not afraid of being stressed.

- Stress helps me remember what is most important in my life.
- Stress keeps me focused on my goals.
- I do not let this stress consume me.
- I manage my stress in healthy and productive ways.
- I have the main control over the stress that I feel. No one else is in charge of my feelings.
- It is normal for me to be peaceful.
- I allow this lifestyle to take over every aspect, making it easier to have a more relaxed sleep.
- When I can truly calm myself down all the way, it will be easier to stay asleep.
- I let go of my anxiety because it serves me no purpose.
- I am excited for the future.
- I am not afraid of any of the challenges that I might face.
- It is easy for me to be more and more relaxed.
- There is nothing more freeing than realizing that I do not have to be anxious over certain aspects in my life.
- I will sleep easier and more peacefully knowing that there is nothing in this world that I need to be afraid of.
- Nothing feels better than crawling into my bed after a long day.
- My bedroom is filled with peace and serenity. I have no trouble drifting off to sleep.
- Everything in my room helps me to be more relaxed.

- I feel safe and at peace knowing that I am protected in my room.
- I have no trouble falling asleep once I am able to close my eyes and focus on my breathing.
- I make sure all of my anxieties are gone so that I can fall asleep easier.
- When bad thoughts come into my head, I know how to push them away so that I can focus instead on getting a better night's sleep.
- I am centered on reality, which involves getting the best sleep possible.
- It is so refreshing to wake up after a night of rest that was uninterrupted.
- Any time that I might wake up, I have no trouble knowing how to get myself back to sleep.
- Whenever I wake up, it is easy to get out of bed within the first few times that my alarm clock rings.
- The better night's sleep I get, the easier it is for me to wake up.
- I release all of the times that I have had a restless night's sleep.
- No matter how many times I have struggled with my sleep in the past, I know that I am capable of getting the best night's sleep possible.
- My sleep history doesn't matter now. I want to get a good night's sleep, so I will.
- The more I focus on falling and staying asleep, the fresher I will feel in the morning.

- Getting a good night's sleep helps me look better as well. My hair is bouncier, my face is fresher, my eyes are wider, and my smile is bigger.
- Sleep is something that I need.
- Sleep is something that I deserve.
- No matter how little work I got done in a day, or how much more I might have to do the next day, I need to get sleep.
- There is no point in my life where sleep would be entirely bad for me. It's like drinking water. I could always at least use a little bit of it.
- I am alert when I am focused on sleeping better.
- It is easier to remember the important things I need to keep stored in my memory when I have been able to have a full night's sleep.
- I can focus on what is going on around me more when I have been able to sleep through the night.
- There is nothing about getting sleep that is bad for me. As long as I am doing it in a healthy way, it will improve my life.
- I know how to cut out bad sleeping habits.
- I understand what is important to start doing to get a better sleep.
- As soon as I start to lay down, I am focused on drifting away.
- I do not let anxious thoughts keep me awake anymore.
- I will sleep healthy from here on out because I know that it is one of the most important decisions for my health that I can make.

- I'm not afraid of fear. Fear does not control me. In fact, fear is merely a reaction.
- I choose consciously to let go of my past worries and to move forward into the good and the light that await me.
- I am strong and capable. I grow stronger with every breath I take, and every time I exhale, my fears leave me.
- I reject failure, and I choose to fill my mind and soul with only positive nurturing thoughts.
- I believe that I can, and, therefore, I believe if not today, tomorrow I will succeed.
- I am like a magnet. I repel negativity and negative thoughts in all forms.
- I do not make mistakes, but rather I learn lessons - and from every lesson I have learned more and more.
- I am willing to invest in my power to change my life by releasing the anxiety that holds me back.
- I am stronger than I may seem.
- My fears and my depression do not control who I am or who I am going to be.
- I am on a constant journey to discover a more calm and peaceful version of me.
- I have made it through this far, and I will make it through until the end.
- I belong exactly where I am. I am not unwanted or ugly – I am perfection.

- I celebrate everything that has to do with me, because I am madly in love with myself and all that I can be.
- I will love myself enough to get through this moment.
- I choose to feel safe and secure, even when the darkness comes in.
- Anxiety is a real problem, but I am a real solution and my mind is stronger than anxiety's grip on it.
- Anxiety does not control me; it merely shows me where not to go and what not to do.
- Anxiety is merely the fear of the unknown, and I am an explorer who is ready to know everything.
- I have survived this far, and I will survive as long as I want.
- I am someone who is capable of looking beyond the pain that has been inflicted upon me, because pain does not matter, and what I choose to do does matter.
- I am whole despite my anxiety.
- My anxiety cannot control me, because I do not allow it to be in the driving seat.
- I have everything I need to be the best version of me.
- I am always in charge of my own mind, l, and my mind does not choose to be anxious.

## 23. Love and Marriage Affirmations

The best way to receive love, it to first give love. And the best way to be surrounded by loving people, it to first become a loving person. Why choose love instead of hate? Well, hate is too big of a burden to bear as Martin Luther King, Jr. put it. Love is powerful as it has the power to turn an enemy into a friend. But to express true love towards anyone else in your life, you must first love the most important person in your life which is you! You are incredibly complex, and there's no one with the exact same DNA and brain configuration as you. You have talents, abilities and inclinations that are unique to you and the best way to serve the world and people around you is use them in a positive way. So, love yourself for who you are, and you'll find that loving others will become second nature. Here are affirmations about loving yourself, loving others and loving the world we live in.

- I love the world and all its beauty.
- God's love is circulating in my life as well as flows to me in avalanches of abundance.
- I understand that I'm the only one who can be me and that I was made this way for a reason.
- The world will be a better place because I was here.
- I choose love, forgiveness and kindness.
- I love myself and all the goods deeds I have made and will make.
- I see loving eyes all around me.
- I deserve to experience love.

- I get love in abundance.
- I give love and I receive love.
- Every day and in every way, I'm choosing to look at life through a lens of love.
- My life is now full of love as I have attracted the most loving person into my life.
- I have the perfect partner and our love is incredibly strong.
- I am a wonderful, trustworthy and understanding person.
- I attract wonderful, trustworthy and understanding people into my life.
- I forgive myself and others.
- I do small things for others to show my love for them.
- I radiate true love to my partner.
- My partner radiates true love to me.
- I give love freely and effortlessly.
- I am open to receive love from the Universe.
- I am open to receive love from other people.
- I am an exceptional giver, and I'm also an exceptional receiver.
- I am surrounded by other people who love and care for me.
- I live in a loving and caring Universe.
- I support my friends and family.
- I attract relationships that are of pure and unconditional love.

- I look at the good in life, and I see love all around me.
- I am so happy and peaceful now that I've found the love within me.
- I live in a romantic relationship with the partner of my dreams.
- I love my healthy body.
- I love my brain and all its abilities.
- I find it easy to admire others and show appreciation.
- I am super confident and other people are very attracted to my confidence.
- I am being guided by a loving universe.
- Love is my birthright and always find opportunities to experience love.
- I am so grateful for having the most wonderful and loving partner in my life.
- I acknowledge the good in others and make fault seem easy to correct.
- I am an excellent and loving leader and others are naturally attracted to my being.
- My mind, heart and soul work in perfect harmony to create love all the time.
- My efforts are being supported by a loving Universe.
- I only need my own approval.
- I trust myself and my ability to make the right choices.

- I trust my gut feeling and intuition to guide me to an ever-loving destination.
- I accept others as they are and in turn the accept me for who I am.
- My mind contains loving thoughts about myself and others.
- I attract love easily and effortlessly.
- I am worthy of feeling self-love and a love for others.
- I am love.
- I now live in a beautiful state filled with abundance and love.
- I am so happy with the person I am with.
- I love and respect my partner so much.
- I compliment and show affection for my partner.
- I am caring and harmonious.
- I am calm and easy to work with.
- My partner is wonderful, and I reward them for that.
- My partner takes time to show their affection for me.
- My partner listens to me.
- I listen to my partner.
- Time flows easily when I am with my partner.
- My partner completes me.
- I reinforce the things I like about my partner.
- My partner is madly in love with me.

- My partner and I have great sex.
- I am extremely attracted to my partner.
- I love so many things about my partner.
- I have so much gratitude for getting to be with my partner.
- My relationship is awesome.
- In my relationship I get to do what I want and have a great partner.
- I have such a great partner.
- I have a wonderful and thoughtful partner.
- My relationship is getting better and better.
- Every day, I find myself loving my partner more and more.
- I love the person I am with all of the time, no matter what.
- My partner is fantastic in a multitude of ways.
- I have great love in my life.
- My relationship is strong.
- I love my relationship.
- Communication is great in my relationship.
- I communicate with my partner effectively, and without issue.
- I try to point out what's good about my partner.
- I make my partner feel valued, loved, and respected.
- I am generous with my partner.

- My relationship is a source of joy in my life.
- My relationship is good enough.
- Our relationship makes both of us happy.
- I use compliments instead of complaints with my partner.
- I communicate in a calm and friendly manner with my partner.
- My partner makes me happy, and joyous.
- I expect my partner to be human, and not perfect.
- I forgive my partner for their mistakes and errors.
- My partner and I are in love.
- I tell my partner how important they are every day.
- I make my partner feel valued, and important.
- My partner is important to me, and I love them.
- I love my partner and am as pleasant as possible with them.
- My life is so great with my partner.
- I love being with my partner, and I tell them that every day.
- Everything will work out well with my partner.
- My partner is great.
- I love my partner.
- I express my love to my partner all the time.
- I try to change myself before changing others.
- I keep my emotions under my rule.

- I choose what to say with minimal reactivity.
- I have a wonderful relationship.
- I love who I am with at all times.
- The person I am with is wonderful.
- I am so glad to have the partner that I do.
- I love to spend time with my partner.
- I always tell my partner how important they are.
- I always tell my partner how important they are to me.
- I enthusiastically tell my partner all the things they do right.
- I am responsible for my happiness; my partner is someone to share my happiness with.
- I am responsible for all things in my life.
- My partner and I live abundantly together.
- I always tell my partner when they do something right.
- I try to catch my partner doing the right thing.
- I treat my partner like the important person that they are at all times.
- I love so many things about the person I am with.
- I expect my partner to make mistakes and forgive them.
- My partner is so supporting and loving.
- My partner cheers me up all the time.
- My partner is there for me when I need them most.

- My partner is happy.
- My partner is a very happy person.
- My partner is very romantic.
- My partner is very thoughtful.
- My partner loves and respects me.
- My partner respects my space, time, and ideas.
- I have such a loving and caring partner.
- I love the relationship I am in so much.
- I am so happy and grateful for how awesome my partner is.
- My life with my partner is amazing.
- I love how great my life is with my partner.
- My relationship is getting stronger every day.
- I love how my partner looks.
- I love how my partner talks.
- I love how in tune my partner is with my thoughts.
- I love the person I am with, and they love me.
- My relationship is always growing stronger and stronger.
- My life is so great and wonderful.
- I love spending time with my partner.
- I love watching movies and tv with my partner.
- I love my partner every day of the year.

- I am falling deeper in love day after day.
- My relationship is absolutely amazing.
- My partner brightens my life and raises my happiness.
- My partner is so good at getting stuff done.
- My partner is an awesome person.
- I feel so lucky for getting to be with my partner.
- My partner turns me on so much.
- I get so horny for my partner.
- My partner and I both help each other out.
- My partner and I are an unstoppable team.
- My partner is amazing in so many departments.
- I thrive with my partner.
- My partner and I are champions in our industries.
- My partner and I have strong life purposes.
- I love my partner so much, and all the things they do for me.
- I love looking deep into my partner's eyes.
- I trust my partner more and more each day.
- I know my partner loves me to the end of the earth.
- I feel so much love right now for my partner.
- My life is like a dream come true.
- My partner makes my world so happy.

- My happiness is fully my responsibility.
- My partner is such a fun and happy person.
- My partner is always making me more and more abundant.
- My partner is always making me happier and happier.
- My partner and I have so much money.
- My partner and I have more and more passive income each year.
- My partner and I take lavish vacations together.
- My partner and I accomplish so much great work together.
- I am with the most amazing person in the world; I feel so lucky!
- My partner is such a great and joyous part of my life.

# 24. Success and Wealth Affirmations

What is a successful mind? Well it's a mind that contains positive and empowering beliefs about success regarding all aspects of life. It has been said that people fear success more than failure, and with that mindset, it is hard to achieve anything extraordinary. The affirmations below will not only help you overcome any subconscious blocks that might be holding you back from living your dreams, but they will also prime your mind to spot any wealth creating opportunities and more importantly; encourage you to act on them.

- My beliefs shape my reality.
- I realize that I'm the creator of my life.
- I decide to make my life a masterpiece.
- I know that if I believe it I can see it.
- I have always been destined to become wealthy.
- I find a lot of opportunities for creating prosperity and abundance.
- I give and receive.
- I live by the words "let go and grow". That's why I find it easy to forgive myself and others.
- I'm grateful for the lessons my past has given me.
- I'm a great giver; I'm also a great receiver.
- I understand that my abundance of money can make the world a better place.

- The universe responds to my mindset of abundance by giving me more prosperity.
- I define my dream and feel gratitude for its realization.
- I visualize living my dream every day.
- I send out good vibrations about money.
- I'm abundant in every way.
- I'm grateful for all the money that I have. I'm grateful for all the prosperity that I receive.
- I'm grateful for the present moment and focus on the beauty of life.
- I pay myself first and make my money multiply.
- I have a millionaire mind and I now understand the principles behind wealth.
- I love the freedom that money gives me.
- I'm a multi-millionaire.
- I choose to be me and free.
- There is an infinite amount of opportunities for creating wealth in the world.
- I see opportunities for creating wealth and act on them.
- My motto is act and adapt.
- The answers always seem to come to me.
- I have an attitude of gratitude.
- I deserve to become wealthy.

- I deserve to have the best in life.
- I'm a wonderful person with patience.
- I trust the universe to guide me to my true calling in life. Knowing this I get a feeling of calmness.
- I know that I'm becoming the best I can possibly be.
- I feel connected to prosperity.
- I love money and realize all the great things it can do.
- I'm at one with a tremendous amount of money.
- Money loves me and therefore it will keep flowing to me.
- I use my income wisely and always have a big surplus of money at the end of the month.
- I truly love the feeling of being wealthy. I enjoy the freedom it gives me.
- It is easy for me to understand how money works.
- I choose to think in ways that support me in my happiness and success.
- I'm an exceptional manager of money.
- I realize that success in anything leaves clues.
- I follow the formula of people who have created a fortune.
- I create a lot value for others.
- I'm a valuable person.
- My life is full of abundance.

- I know about the 80 20 rule which states that 80 % of the effects come from 20 % of the causes.
- 20 % of my activities produce 80 % of the results.
- I choose to focus on the most important things in my life.
- I choose to become wealthy.
- I make my money multiply by investing them wisely.
- I pay myself first. 10 % of my income works for me.
- I increase my ability to earn by setting concrete goals and work to achieve them.
- By implementing the 80 20 rule in my life I increase my productivity and profitability.
- I focus on the most important areas in my life and eliminate, delegate or automate the rest.
- Time is on my side now.
- Everyday I'm getting better, smarter and more skillful.
- I believe that other people want me to be successful and are happily helping me towards my dream.
- I know how to handle people.
- I smile often and remember the other person's name.
- I give sincere appreciation and focus on the other person.
- I make people feel important.
- I praise improvement and call attention to people's mistakes indirectly. I make fault seem easy to correct.

- I'm a great leader and people are happy about doing what I suggest.
- I'm a good listener who encourages the other person to talk about him or herself.
- I try honestly to see things from the other persons view.
- I cooperate with others; whose minds work in perfect harmony for the attainment of a common definite objective.
- I have a purpose and a plan.
- I'm courageous and understand that courage is not the absence of fear but rather the willingness to act in spite of it.
- I have self discipline and full control over my thoughts and emotion.
- I do the most important things first.
- I'm organized and remember the 80 20 rule.
- I expect the best in life. I know about the magic of thinking big.
- I always expect to win.
- I'm a confident person who takes action.
- I'm decisive and know what I want.
- I'm committed to my success.
- I know that where attention goes energy flows.
- I see opportunities and act on them.
- I write down my goals and program my subconscious mind for success.

- I will persist until I succeed.
- I only pray for guidance and I realize that I'm going to be tested.
- I get stronger by challenges.
- I live everyday as if it was my last.
- I realize that life is a gift.
- I'm grateful for being alive.
- I understand that being born is a miracle and I'm very grateful for it.
- I'm more than I seem to be and all the powers of the universe are within me.
- I feel abundance and love.
- I trust myself; my gut feeling knows the truth.
- I harness my intuition and know that people might be like me, but that I'm unique.
- My DNA and the way my brain is configured is completely unique.
- I love myself and understand that I'm the only one who can be me.
- I focus on my inclinations and the things I'm good at.
- I develop my talents and abilities.
- I focus on adding value.
- The world will be a better place because I was here.
- I'm a valuable person who takes responsibility.

- I get success in all that I do
- I easily achieve my goals
- I have absolute faith in my success Success is mine to be enjoyed
- I have everything I need to succeed
- I am living my dream
- I am experiencing fantastic success
- Success and good fortune flow towards me in a river of abundance
- I attract success and prosperity with all of my ideas
- Success and achievement are natural outcomes for me
- All of my thoughts, plans, and ideas Lead me straight to success
- Prosperity and success is my natural state of mind
- I Ascend to the top of Corporate ladder and my salary stop the charts
- My management skills open the door of opportunities
- I am the example of success and triumph

# 25. Signaling the Universe Through Gratitude

When people first learn about the Law of Attraction and the immense power of their thoughts, their first question is often about how to communicate with the Universe in a way that will guarantee they attract good things instead of bad ones.

And the best answer for accomplishing this always comes down to GRATITUDE.

If the only new habit you ever added to your life was gratitude, you'd already have everything you needed to begin manifesting the life that you love. Thinking about the things you're grateful for each and every day is one of the most powerful practices you can ever do. And if you could only just stop worrying about what isn't here yet, and start appreciating what is, everything in your life would turn around and improve.

Every time you say, "I'm grateful for that." or "I appreciate that." or "I really like that." -- you're moving energy and creating space for more of what you like to be pulled in toward you. It's universal law. This is especially effective because it's impossible to appreciate one thing and worry about something else at the same time. So every second spent in gratitude (of anything at all) is also a moment spent drawing whatever you want toward you, rather than inviting what you don't want instead.

More than most any other positive emotion out there, gratitude is the key to truly manifesting your desires because of the message that feeling automatically broadcasts to the Universe.

You see, when you simply "wish" for something, you're actually pushing it away from you. This is because the act of "wishing" only reaffirms energetically that you don't have it, which then instantly instructs the Universe to keep it away from you. Gratitude, on the other hand, affirms a state of being in which your desire has already been given to you -- which then automatically draws that desire into your manifested physical reality.

If the only thing you did every day was feel grateful more often than you felt any negative emotion at all, everything in your life would improve. Your health, your finances, your relationships -- everything! This paragraph may very well be the most important thing you read in this, so don't just gloss over it.

This is the key to everything!

The best part is that once you have a little practice under your belt, feeling genuine gratitude for even the smallest things in your life becomes very easy (and very enjoyable) to do. And before you know it, you're manifesting things you've waited years for.

This is why gratitude is so powerful. And this is why it's one of the best things to have in your life each and every day.

And since feeling gratitude is such a simple, easy, AND enjoyable thing to do, there's absolutely NO reason why it shouldn't be a daily part of your life.

## The Key To Feeling Gratitude

(How To Actually "Do It")

Gratitude is a core human emotion that's very easy to access.

There's no trick to it. If you're worried for any reason that you're not "doing it right", that might just be another case of the ego doing its best to keep things the way they are. But there's no "how" to actually worry about. You just do it.

Even so, if you still need a little more guidance anyway, an easy method for experiencing gratitude is to think of something you have right now that you don't want to lose. And whatever it is - think of the reasons why you want to keep it. ...Whatever those reasons are, it's impossible to consider them without also feeling appreciation for the thing that you're thinking about. You're brought directly into a state of gratitude because you're now recognizing why these things are so valuable to you, why you want them, and therefore, why you're grateful to have them. Simple as that.

Can't think of anything off the top of your head? How about your paycheck. The clothes you're wearing. The roof over your head. The food you eat.. A pleasant memory that brings a smile to your face. How about the air in your lungs. The last time someone did a favor for you. The last time you laughed out loud. Your bed that keeps you warm and comfortable every night. Your amazing heart that literally beats NONSTOP to distribute nutrients to other vital organs that are also working tirelessly for you. There's SO MUCH to be grateful for. I barely scratched the surface. I

I do, however, want to remind you that it's also possible to feel gratitude even when you're faced with undesirable circumstances.

For example, it might seem difficult to appreciate where you're living if you dislike your neighbors. But that roof and those walls still keep you warm in the winter, cool in the summer, and dry any time it ever rains. And no matter how much you might not like your job or your boss, that paycheck you're getting is still the reason you get to eat every day. And it's keeping you afloat while you figure out a way to get a better job (which is WAY more possible than you've been allowing yourself to realize until now).

One of the methods you'll read in the next few pages actually leverages the things in your life that don't please you, and shows you how to turn the situation around immediately, experience gratitude that very instant, and finally begin attracting all the things you've ever wanted. Another method will give you the opportunity to attract future events into your life with the same level of certainty that you have for things that are already here.

All of them will be useful. But none will be required. So try them. Test them. Play around with them. Experiment. See which ones feel the best. Do them in a way that fits your schedule. The instructions will be clear and direct, but there's always enough flexibility to modify them in simple ways to make them your own. For example, if it doesn't feel natural to begin a sentence with the words "I'm so happy and grateful now that…", you can begin with "I'm very happy that…" or "I'm thankful that…" or "Thank you for…" or whatever else fits in with how you naturally speak.

The bottomline is that these are powerful in a way that I could never describe in just words. So dive in. And have fun.

# 26. Manifestation Methods

## The Stacking Method

The Gratitude Stacking Method for manifesting your desires is as simple and direct as they come. It's also a great exercise to do if you don't have a lot of time.

Step 1: Write out a list of things you're grateful for.

Step 2: Read through each item on your list.

Step 3: As you're reading them -- one at a time -- take 20-60 seconds (however long you personally prefer) to really feel the gratitude of whatever you're describing.

Feel free to write down anything that gives you a feeling of gratitude. It can be a material possession that you own. It could be an event that you enjoyed. It could be a fun memory of someone or something. Let your imagination soar and add anything that you're inspired to.

When you go through each "item" on your list, say it out loud if you're alone. But if you're in a public place, and you don't want to attract unwanted attention, you can just read it in your head instead.

As for how long this should take you, it's really up to you since you decide how big you want your list to be. You might have 10 things, or just 5, or if you're really in a rush -- you might only write 3 things that day.

Whatever you put down, you can list things that have happened in the past, things you have now, or even things that you wish to have in the future.

Regardless of "when" each thing occurred, it should always be phrased in the PRESENT tense (even future events), and begin with wording similar to:

"I'm so happy and grateful for…"

"I'm so happy and grateful now that…"

"I'm so thankful now that…"

"I'm so excited now that…"

"I'm grateful for…"

It's called the 'stacking' method because you're stacking a bunch of things on top of one another in one big list of gratitude. The name also invites you to write larger lists when you have the time for them since a list with more items helps you get more momentum each time you do a session. The more you pile on, the better you feel.

The purpose of this method is simple: Regardless of whether your list is big or small, this serves as an easy way to guarantee you at least do SOMETHING every day to express gratitude and raise your vibration without it feeling inconvenient or being too time-consuming.

After all, ANYONE can take 60 seconds out to write a few things they're grateful for no matter how busy their schedule is. But ten minutes is even better if they can spare it. And since you get to decide how many things you're going to write, you can be as thorough as you want to without it feeling rushed.

After you give yourself enough practice with this, you'll begin to experience deeper and more profound feelings of gratitude.

You won't have to 'force' them (nor should you ever try to).

They'll just come.

When you do begin to experience it more deeply, it may feel like a warm buzzing in your solar plexus. Or it may feel like you're taking easier calmer breaths. Or your skin might tingle a little. Or you might simply notice yourself experiencing a moment of peace and tranquility.

There's no "one" way that it might happen, there's no one way it HAS to happen, and there's no way to predict how you'll specifically experience it for yourself. So don't worry about getting yourself up to some pre-established "level" of gratitude in order for things to begin manifesting. Just know that the method is working (it is!).

Give it a try next time you have a few minutes to add some gratitude to your day, and have fun.

And yes, it's THAT simple.

## The Time-Lapse Method

This method is basically a gratitude "stack" that includes the same number of past, present, and future things -- but all jumbled in a random order so that the future ones aren't all at the end of the list.

This is one of the very first techniques I teach anyone who's looking to make dramatic changes in their life without any struggle, stress, or confusion. Not only is it extremely simple to use, but once you give yourself a few sessions to really test it out, you'll see that it can be really fun as well.

The most amazing thing about the Time-Lapse Method is how easily it magnetizes your vibrational setpoint for things you want that haven't occurred yet. It does this by taking the same certainty and confidence you have for things that have already happened for you (or are currently happening for you now), and directly applies that identical certainty and confidence to future events as well.

You're technically doing this to your 'vibration' and not your actual state of belief since, it's WAY easier to instantly alter your vibration (or state of being) moment by moment.

But the beauty of this is that over a period of time, your beliefs will also eventually adjust to your new desired reality on their own without you having to force them to.

Your best bet for getting the most out of this exercise is to make sure you're stacking at least 15 different things that you're grateful for. Begin by writing a list of:

- At least 5 "things" you've had in your past
- At least 5 "things" you have in your present
- At least 5 "things" you want to have in your future.

A "thing" could be a physical object, a goal you achieved (or want to achieve), an event you experienced (or want to experience), or anything else positive that has happened in your life (or will happen). Regardless of whether they're past events, current events, or future events -- for each of them, use statements that express gratitude in the PRESENT tense.

Once your list is complete, mix it up so that it's not in chronological order anymore. For example:

1. Present thing/event
2. Past thing/event
3. Future thing/event
4. Present thing/event
5. Past thing/event
6. Present thing/event
7. Future thing/event
8. Future thing/event
9. Past thing/event

10. Future thing/event
11. Present thing/event
12. Past thing/event
13. Past thing/event
14. Future thing/event
15. Present thing/event

Once your list is ready, read through every item one at a time (out loud if you're alone, or in your head if you're in public). As you go through each, take 20-60 seconds (however long you personally prefer) to really feel the gratitude of whatever you're describing.

To give you a little more clarity on this, let's say for example:

-you CURRENTLY are making $90,000 per year

-you FOUND your perfect apartment 3 years ago, and you're still happy living there

-you WANT TO be promoted to Vice President of the company you work for

-you CURRENTLY are in a happy committed relationship

In this situation, if you're using the sample order as above, the first four statements on your gratitude list might be stated on the following way (all present tense):

1. "I'm so happy and grateful to be making $90,000 a year."
2. "Thank you for the perfect apartment I found that I'm still happily living in."
3. "I'm so grateful for my promotion to Vice President of my company."

4. "I'm so happy and grateful that I'm in such a happy and committed relationship."

This may seem simple, but it is VERY, VERY POWERFUL.

The reason this method is so effective is because most of what's on your list are things that have already manifested in your actual reality. So when you go through those past and present manifestations, there's a "certainty" in your vibration that carries over and applies to the 'future' statements as well.

It's simply easier and more natural for your body to regulate your emotions by not letting them stray too far from one another in such a brief period of time without an external stimuli triggering them.

So now, rather than having to worry about reprogramming your beliefs in order to get what you want (which many people find extremely difficult), you'll instead be using a very simple (and easy) technique to set your vibration up as if you already do believe that what you want is yours!

This signal of "having it" is being transmitted to both your subconscious mind AND the Universe in its entirety without any resistance.

In summary, by jumbling past, present, and future manifestations up, you're basically "tricking" your vibration into setting a more potent and robust point of attraction -- one that you wouldn't be able to do as easily if you were only focusing on future events.

This method is fun, it's easy, and IT WORKS.

## Gratitude Attraction Boosters

While the Stack and Time-Lapse methods are extremely potent on their own, there are also a few fun and easy strategies (or "attraction boosters") that you can use to amplify your feelings of gratitude and shift your vibrational point of attraction even faster.

These are so easy to do that many people automatically add all of them to every gratitude session they do.

Boost Option #1: Saying 'Thank You' at the end of your session.

As you're finishing up your list of things that you're grateful for, simply tack on a "thank you, Universe, for giving this to me." at the end of it (or any similar message that makes sense with what you had listed).

You can swap the word "Universe" out with "Infinite Intelligence", "higher self", "inner being", "God", "universal consciousness" ...or anything else that feels right for you and helps amplify the appreciation that you're experiencing in that moment.

Through this extra 'thank you' in advance, you're reaffirming your confidence in what's on the way to you more deeply, which stirs your feelings of positivity even more, and energetically shifts things even further in your favor. If you want to, you can even enhance the experience by visualizing "someone" (or really, some 'being') in front of you to thank.

You might imagine a warm outline of glowing energy in the shape of a human body.

Or you might see a cloud or mist of light. This "being" can be in the room with you or looking down from the stars.

There's no wrong way of doing it as long as it feels good and is amplifying your experience.

Feel free to say "thank you" more than once if it helps. Say it 5 times. 10 times. 100 times. Whatever you prefer. Try it once, and you'll understand how helpful it really is.

Boost Option #2: Saying WHY You're Grateful For Each Thing

As you list each thing that you're grateful for, feel free to include reasons why you're grateful.

It's certainly effective enough to say "I'm so happy and grateful for my new promotion." But you can instantly boost it by going deeper and saying "I'm so happy and grateful for my new promotion because the extra pay is adding so much more comfort to my life, the bigger office with the extra large windows lets so much sunlight in and really keeps me in a good mood, and my new assigned parking space means I no longer need to interrupt what I'm doing every morning to make sure the meter is fed."

If you have the time to include it in your daily routine, this option really helps make every session more robust and enjoyable, and it also helps give you something more to look forward to the next day.

Boost Option #3: Mentally Directing Your Gratitude Out Through Your Heart

As you read through each item in your gratitude list (and as you do Boost Option #1), amplify the power and feeling of your appreciation by imagining your gratitude vibrating outward from the center of your chest as a ray of brilliant warm light. The light can be white, gold, or any bright color that feels good.

This light is your way of offering positivity, love, and even healing energy to the entire Universe around you. You're thanking everything around you for making things better ...by making things better for everything around you. You'll be amazed at how much more thankful you naturally feel as you do this.

All 3 boosters are convenient, effective, and fun. Give them a shot and see for yourself.

## The Blitz Method

Whether you're writing it down, saying it out loud, or even just thinking it in your mind, Gratitude Blitzing is one of the healthiest and most enjoyable ways to raise your vibration, improve your mood, and attract amazing things into your life.

The Blitz Method is simply the process of listing out a large number of different things to be grateful for, one after another, without any breaks. You can do this for either a specific period of time or until your list reaches a specific minimum number of things. This is all about experiencing a nonstop barrage of gratitude and feelings of appreciation that gain momentum, build on themselves with every passing second, and help you achieve a highly attractive and receptive state very quickly and easily. If you base your Blitz on time, you should engage in the process a minimum of 60-90 seconds. But many people have so much fun with this, they often get themselves up to 5 or even 10 minutes at a time with only a little practice. If you base it on a minimum number of "items," you should come up with a list of at least 25-30 things. But lots of people enjoy making even bigger lists of at least 100 different items.

There's lots of ways of doing this effectively. You can choose a specific topic or theme (such as your body, your health, your finances, etc.). Or you can even just list out whatever comes to mind without worrying whether anything you say relates to anything else you've already put down. How easy is it to come up with a list? Just begin and see how far you can go. You'll be pleasantly surprised once you realize you can list ANYTHING as long as you're grateful for it.

You can have gratitude for the air in your lungs, the roof over your head, the clothes on your back, the fact that you eat every day, your access to clean water, your access to warm water, your access to running water, every dollar in your bank account, your most recent paycheck, your strong healthy heart, your arms, your hands, your fingers, your legs, your feet, your toes, your eyes, your ears, your kidneys, your brain, your liver, your skin, every organ that functions perfectly without you having to think about it, your favorite shirt, your favorite shoes, pizza, pancakes, roller coasters, cool autumns, holidays, snowballs, sunny skies, your best friend from the second grade, ice cream, cookies, your favorite song, hot stone massages, your first kiss, your NEXT kiss, a warm hug from someone you love, this paragraph right now, the fact that you can read it, the fact that you can afford to buy this, birthday cakes, birthday parties, costume parties, the first time you fell in love, the first time you had a crush on someone, the first time someone had a crush on you, the money on the way to you right now, the success you're going to achieve in the next few months, all the people that have been there for you in your life, all the favors they've ever done for you, that smile from a stranger across the room, working electricity, toothpaste, kung fu movies, comic books, professional wrestling, friendly dogs, cotton candy, popcorn, supermarkets, farmers markets, theme parks, apple pie, pumpkin pie, cherry pie, spring breaks, summers at the beach, your first party, funny videos, socks with Star Wars characters on them, your favorite tv show, video games, your favorite cartoon growing up, your first concert, your first car, high speed internet, the last time you smiled, the last time you laughed, the last time you cheered, your phone, your computer, animal crackers, email, refrigerators, cupcakes, cereal boxes with prizes inside, and on and on.

THAT'S how easy it is to list things to be grateful for.

OPTIONAL POWER BOOST: If you want an easy way to amplify this experience, make sure to note WHY you're grateful for each item as you list it out. It takes longer, but it also fires a lot more neurons in your brain. Either way, you can't lose.

At the very end of your blitz, say "thank you!" out loud (or in your head, if you're in public) with as much emotion and appreciation as you can. Say it 3 times ...or even 7 times ...or even 20 times ...or just keep saying it over and over and over and over again for at least one full minute: "Thank you, thank you, thank you, thank you, thank you thank you, Thank You, Thank You, Thank You, Thank You!, Thank You!!, Thank You!!, THANK YOU!, THANK YOU!, THANK YOU!, THANK YOU!!!!, THANK YOU!!!!, THANK YOU!!!!!!!!!!!!"

# 27. How to Live a Happy Life Everyday

Have you ever asked yourself, "How can I live a happy life every day?" Is it even really possible? Is there really a technique or strategy on how to live a happy life every day? Or is there a principle or law that we can follow to live a happy life every day?

I'll share a few techniques and tips on how to really live a happy life every day.

One of the best books I've read about happiness is Being Happy, by Andrew Matthews.

What I really like about the book is that it tackles more about the human mind. The human mind can be compared to an iceberg.

The tip of the iceberg, which we can see, is the conscious part of the brain. The bigger part of the iceberg, which we don't usually see, is the subconscious.

The subconscious mind is the quiet part of the brain which records our thoughts, habits, memories, and which also influences our actions. More often than not, the things we experience in life, especially the behaviors that keep coming back, are caused by the subconscious mind.

You may be thinking, "So, Andrian, what does that have to do with our happiness?"

Well, in order to live a happy life every day, we need to put happy, positive, nurturing, inspirational, and motivational thoughts into our conscious and subconscious mind. Some of you may be asking, "Andrian, how can I do that?"

Here are the 6 Ways to Live a Happy Life Every Day:

1. Gratitude

One of the secrets of the happiest people I know is that they are always thankful for everything they have, whether they have it in abundance or not.

Anthony Robbins once said, "The antidote to fear is gratitude. The antidote to anger is gratitude. You can't feel fear or anger while feeling gratitude at the same time."

Yes, being filled with gratitude for everything can really have a great impact on our lives. Why? Because once we feel grateful for everything, we will naturally feel good.

Try this simple technique right now: Think of three things which you are grateful for right this moment. For example, your smartphone, the Internet, the food you eat, or even the clothes you are wearing right now. Say "thank you" for them. Doesn't that feel good? Yup, it does!

So my advice is that when you feel sad, discouraged, angry, or any other negative feeling, try to think about the things you are grateful for and your mind will wander to other good, positive things in your life. You will definitely feel better.

2. Forgiveness

Mahatma Gandhi once said, "The weak can never forgive. Forgiveness is the attribute of the strong."

Are you strong? Do you hold a grudge in your heart toward someone? Is it really difficult for you to forgive?

Yes, I know it's difficult and really hard to do. But do you know when you're not forgiving, you're only hurting yourself over and over again, while the one who has hurt you is maybe sitting on the beach, enjoying life, and totally clueless about the pain and hurt you feel?

So, now, "let's be STRONG," as Mahatma Gandhi stated above. You may be thinking, "Andrian, I want to forgive. I want to be strong. I just don't know how to forgive. How do I do that?"

I'm going to tell you a simple technique that I've been using for years.

Forgiveness takes place in your mind. There is no need for you to go personally to someone to forgive him or her. You can do it right here, right now, using only your mind.

Once someone has done something to me that's not good or that I've been hurt by, and it keeps on repeating over and over again in my mind, this is what I do:

I close my eyes and imagine the person who has wronged me as if I'm talking to him face to face. I say, "I'm hurt by what you said/did (be specific), but I know you said/did that because (try to look at their perspective as objectively as you can). I would like to say I'm sorry if I've done something to offend you. Today, right now, I'm choosing to forgive you. I'm now forgiving you. I'm now releasing you. And I'm now free. I'm now free."

From then on, my mind is in blessing mode. My mind is now ready to receive peace and blessings. As the Bible says in Romans 12:14, "bless and do not curse." Go ahead and try the technique outlined above and "be strong." You will feel peace and happiness continually come into your life every single day. The more you forgive, the more you'll feel peaceful inside.

You can do this every day, even with the small irritations that come your way. I know this is really effective. Remember, friend, it's all in your mind, so it's better to overcome it in your mind.

3. Love Yourself

Someone once said, "You cannot give what you do not have." I believe that's definitely true. You cannot give an apple to someone if you don't have an apple. You cannot give love to someone if you don't have love to give.

The question now is: "How can we love ourselves?"

Here are some ways we can love ourselves more:

a) Have "me" time. Have time for yourself, alone. No distractions, no social media, no responsibilities, no phones, no calls – just you, alone. During this time, think and reflect on what's happening in your life right now.

Create a strategy. Make a plan to achieve your dreams. Go somewhere quiet where you can think well. Go to the beach. Go for a drive in the country. Go to the mountains. Read a book that inspires you. Just give yourself a break. You deserve it. This will definitely fill up your "love tank."

b) Forgive yourself. Yes, you might stumble sometimes, but learn to forgive yourself. We all make mistakes, and we all fail at times in our lives.

It's not good to be eaten up by guilt, condemnation, or regrets. Forgive yourself. Ask God to forgive you, confess your sins to Him. God says in Proverbs 28:13 (NKJV), "He who covers his sins will not prosper, but whoever confesses and forsakes them will have mercy."

Remember that God is always ready to forgive you, once you ask. So forgive yourself more often, and always say to yourself, "I'm going to do better next time."

c) Do what you love. Remember, you have talents and skills which other people don't have. You are the only person who can do what you can do. So do the things that you love.

Do things which make you feel alive. Follow your passion. If you love writing, then write. If you love dancing, then dance. If you love swimming, then swim. You have your talents and skills for a reason. Use them to nurture the world around you and inspire people.

But most importantly, do it because you love doing it, not because someone else wants you to do it. Have the freedom to live out your passions. Be the best you can be.

d) Grow yourself. Jim Rohn says, "If you want to have more, you have to become more. For things to change, you have to change. For things to get better, you have to get better. For things to improve, you have to improve. If you grow, everything grows for you." He's right!

You need to grow yourself. I know you have dreams and goals. Pursue them. Before you can achieve them, you have to "become more." How? Read books about self-improvement, read the biographies of other successful people, listen to audio/video podcasts that motivate, inspire, and encourage you to become a better person.

Attend seminars and training sessions which cultivate your mind and make you grow. Remember, if you grow, everything grows for you.

Those are just a few ways you can love yourself more. Again, friend, love yourself and live a happy life every day.

4. Associate with Happy and Positive People

As Jack Canfield says, "One of the things I tell people in my seminars is to hang out with positive, nurturing people. You become like who you hang out with."

In order to live a happy life every day, you need to associate yourself with positive, nurturing, happy people. You cannot be with someone who's always complaining, always sad, or always seeing the negative side of things and expect yourself to be happy. Don't allow yourself to be dragged down by the people you associate with.

Find people who are happy and positive, who encourage you and have a deep sense of life. Remember, you always have a choice. Each day you can make a decision about who you will associate with.

If you feel the person you spend most of your time with is dragging you down, or if you feel discouraged or down every time you're with that person, consider this, friend: Their negative attitude may wear off on you. Do you really want that to happen?

Be wise; choose your associates wisely. Always be with happy, positive, and enthusiastic people. These are the people who are there to support you, to encourage you, to motivate you, to inspire you, and to nurture you.

Associate with people who have big dreams, who have a "can-do" attitude, who are optimistic and excited about life, and who have a deep sense of purpose in life.

These are the people who will help you achieve your dreams, who will encourage you when you are down, who will be with you in your success, and who will teach you how to live life.

Choose wisely, friend, and live a happy life every day.

5. Give

One of the best quotes I have ever heard or read is by Anthony Robbins:

"The secret to living is giving."

This is truly one of the secrets to a happy life: giving.

The LORD Jesus Himself said in Acts 20:35, "It is more blessed to give than to receive."

When you give, you naturally feel happy. Because when you give, you produce a chemical in your brain called serotonin which is associated with feeling happy.

In fact, a survey was done of more than 3,000 volunteers of all ages which documented the physical and emotional benefits of giving. A full 50% reported feeling a "helper's high" after helping someone. Other studies have shown that those who give to others experience increased health and happiness.

There you have it, friend. In order to live a happy life every day, give as often as you can. Give to the needy. Give to the poor. Give to charity. Give more to your church, above and beyond your tithe. Give generously.

Proverbs 11:25 states, "A generous person will prosper; whoever refreshes others will be refreshed." So, give more, and live a happy life.

6. Get Enough Restful Sleep

Yes, sleep. That's number six on my list. Why? Because study after study confirms that the more sleep you get, the happier you tend to be. Awesome!

I know, some of us find it extremely hard to get to sleep early; you need to catch up with your favorite TV show, with the news, with the ball game, or you need to socialize with your friends on Facebook, Twitter, Instagram or Pinterest, and so on.

I'm sure you've noticed that the later you go to sleep at night, the harder it is to get up in the morning. And then you're late, so you need to rush through breakfast, getting dressed, and driving to work, only to arrive late at work and have your boss watching you. Then your whole day seems to be hurried, and you feel so negative, like you don't have enough energy. Then after work, you drive back home and do the same thing all over again. This cycle must be stopped! Sleep is the answer. Yes, sleep! Get some rest. Sleep at least 7-8 hours every day. This changes your mood in the morning. You will notice when you have enough restful sleep, you feel invigorated, energized, happy, excited, positive, and overall great. And I assure you your whole day will be great.

So get to sleep early, and live a happy life every day.

There you have it, friend. The six keys to being happy every day. Just as a recap, here they are again:

1. Gratitude
2. Forgiveness
3. Love Yourself
4. Associate with Happy and Positive People
5. Give
6. Get Enough Restful Sleep

Oh, and this is the best part! Did you know there's one ultimate secret to happiness? I've discovered it, and I want to share it with you. For me, this is the greatest secret to happiness:

"My relationship with GOD."

Now, some of you might be saying, "Andrian, you're a religious person, so you have to say that. I'm not religious, and I'd rather not think about such things."

But you know what, friend? This is the real secret to happiness in the world. After I came to know Jesus Christ and surrendered my life to Him, and after I let Him be my LORD and Savior, I've found the true and real meaning of happiness.

This is not about religion. This is about "relationship." You might know about God and maybe even believe in God, but do you have a personal relationship with Him?

A real relationship with God is similar to a relationship with a friend. You have face-to-face conversations and communicate intimately, just like with your friend.

A relationship with God is the same. You can talk to God the same way you talk to your friend. God talks to you through His Word, the Bible, or through another believer, or through the circumstances you're going through.

Friend, always remember that "God loves you."

I believe it's no accident that you are reading this. There's a reason why God put this into your hands: to hear these words, to read these words. You know why, friend?

Because "God loves you."

Friend, if you want to have a personal relationship with God, and you want to surrender everything to Him – your life, your burdens, your problems, your finances, your relationships, your health, whatever it may be – just follow me in this prayer:

"LORD, I know it's not an accident that I am reading this right now. I know there's a reason why You brought me to this point. LORD, I believe my life is meaningless without You. I want to have true peace, true happiness, and true joy in my life. I understand that I can only have that when I'm in a relationship with You. I want that – a personal relationship with You. Today, LORD Jesus, forgive me from all the things I've done, from all my sins and wrongdoings. I repent. I believe in You. I believe You died on the cross for me, to save me so that I may have everlasting life with You. Today, LORD Jesus, I accept You as my LORD and Savior. Starting today, I surrender my life to You and let You take full control. In Jesus' name, Amen."

If you prayed that prayer or something along those lines, "CONGRATULATIONS, FRIEND!" You are now on your journey to true peace, true happiness, and true joy with Jesus Christ. That's the real secret to live a happy life every day.

# 28. How to Calm Your Emotions

## Accept All Emotions

More often, people dealing with depression do not like what they feel, and therefore, they try to avoid anything that brings about emotions. In the short term avoiding these situations and suppressing the emotions is an effective solution in the short term. However, in the long term, the problem becomes bigger than the avoided emotions. In most cases, a depressed individual is affected by negative emotions because it brings about discomfort. Accepting the negative emotions, one is feeling is a sure way of starting to heal from depression. Accepting means being willing to experience the harmful emotions, acknowledging them, and letting them be part of your system; accept that you are sick and give way for the healing process to take place. Through acceptance, you are now able to save the energy that is spent in denying the emotions. To get out of the depression, as an individual, you have already set goals, and having accepted the emotions that are disturbing you, it is will now be easier to keep the behavior that supports your goals.

Accepting all the emotions, helps you to distinguish the harmful emotions and good emotions, use them to your advantage. It will be easier to learn to manage the negative emotions and encourage positive emotions so that they help you experience a positive part of your life.

Accepting all the emotions helps to make them less destructive. It is like a person who fears watching horror movies chooses to watch them until the fear goes away. In the same way, getting used to the emotions would eventually be something normal, and it will have no effect on your moods and interaction with other people. The change will put you on your right foot towards healing.

## Remember that Everything Passes

Something that is causing your depression cannot last forever, and therefore it is good to be optimistic that things will get better. The situation might be hard but focusing on the positive side of the situation would bring a positive impact on your mental well-being, as well as physical. For you to go through the depression and emerge a winner you must be fit mentally and physically, and therefore having positive thinking activates new energy and perspective of looking at issues affecting you. For instance, if it is a financial problem that is causing your depression, it is good to understand that it will come to pass and things will get better. When you tell yourself such words you open up your mind and realize that things will not just happen, you have to do something about it. Consequently, creativity sets in new ideas on how to solve the problems you are facing emerge. The new spirit in you also brings out your best as you develop problem-solving skills and new strategies to cope, knowing that it is just for a short time.

The physical health also improves since you can now manage most of the stressful situation that comes your way, knowing that everything will pass. A healthy body can withstand pain, and resist illness, which lowers the level of stress; imagine a depressed person getting sick more often, it is like adding salt to the injury.

## Depersonalize the Difficulty

Difficulties that are in your way that may come your way do not belong to you, for instance, you do not own poverty, and poverty does not own you. You and the difficulty that you are facing are two different entities that exist alone. This strategy will help you to realize that you can move away from the difficulty because you are not tied together. Therefore, your future does not rely on the difficulty that you are facing, the past experience with the difficulty remains to be just an experience, and what you do to improve your self is what matters. You are the one holding the key to your life, and it is only you who can change it. This helps to align your actions to your goal of healing from depression and becoming a better you.

Depersonalization of the difficulty brings down the emotions that are associated with it, as you do not think of it as part of you. Therefore, it does not affect you emotionally. The control of emotions greatly lowers the symptoms of depression and reduces stress level, and slowly, you will begin to get back to living a normal life. This way, you are able to notice what you feel like a person and what you control, and you cannot. Depersonalizing sometimes is hard, especially if it involves people who are close to you because we fear what they will say, lose our care or help, but you should remember that even if we care for those who are close to us, it is not good to live according to their expectations. It is not your responsibility to care about what other people feel, say, or think, especially, if it causes harm to you or other people. Therefore, if a person makes you feel unsafe, eave the person physically and emotionally, and focus on yourself.

## Change Paradigms

The whole treatment process involves changing your way you think, respond, and even react to situations that disturb you. There is a need to eliminate thoughts about the difficult situation that puts you in a bad mood. Example, thinking that it is your fault that your husband mistreats you is a negative thought that should not be entertained. The thoughts of how to make things better for yourself should now set in, giving you a push towards achieving your goals. The response towards harsh situations that affect our lives should also change, if your spouse died and left you with children, do you cry about if every time children are sent home to collect school fees. This response to the inability to pay for school feel does not solve anything; respond by waking up and looking for a job that helps you pay the fees. You should, therefore, sit down, and evaluate your past thoughts, actions and reactions towards the situation that is causing you depression and check which ones worked to alleviate the situation and which one did not work. Then adopt the ones that worked, and change the ones that worsened or had no effect on the situation. This would help you to get rid of unhealthy thoughts, emotions, actions, and responses, and welcome positive ones. It also enables one to be creative when looking for better strategies to improve the current harmful situation and avoids repeating of mistakes done earlier.

## Surprise Every Wonder

There are things that you wanted to do in life but just wondered if it is possible. To get away from the feeling of depression, you can take up these activities and try executing them; such activities will occupy your mind, making you forget about what depresses you. It is like an adventure, for example, I wonder how birthday cakes are made to look so attractive for the event. Instead of wondering, you take up the initiative to know how it is done and try to bake a birthday cake and decorate it. You can do as many activities as you can to surprise your wonders. The activities might also include taking a tour of your dream city and getting to know more about it. This makes you appreciate things around you, and revives positive thoughts about life; it helps you rethink the situation that is depressing you and bring out statements like, "what if I do things this way, will it be better?" The creativity that will help you get out of the state of depression you are in is also activated, and new ideas are easily conceived. During the execution of the wonderful activities, negative emotions are easily gotten rid of, and positive ones are activated. The activities are also soothing thus helps one to heal mentally and physically.

## Cultivate Gratitude

It is not that everything in your life is negative and is against you. The situation that you are facing is only in a section of your life. Therefore, it is good to appreciate what you have in life. It is good, to begin with, your own life; you are going through tough times, but God has given you a chance to live. This is a reason to show gratitude. One can also cultivate gratitude by engaging in charity work such as helping those who are less fortunate, for example, the poor, old, children living in children homes, and street children, among others. This gesture can make one feel good about himself or herself and start appreciating and loving his or her life. The person starts to realize that he is a good person, and deserves a good treatment and a better life; my life should not be taken for granted. I thank God that I have children, He has given me good health, and why should I languish in depression, and yet there are people who do not have what I have. Gratitude arouses such questions, which brings out positivity, and encourages focus. The person with such an awakening force from inside is likely to align his or her action towards healing from depression. He or she now feels obligated to make his life better. The new energy is good to fight the emotions that cause changes in mood and anxiety.

## Live the Present

When we are faced with situations that are full of uncertainties, staying calm and focusing on what we are doing becomes a problem; this leads to anxiety. Some people are affected more if the future and uncertain events will have a big impact on their life. For example, a teenager who is about to sit for his or her final examination is not able to do the papers well because he or she feels anxious about the outcome of that will decide whether she joins a better school or not. Remember that the future is dependent on the actions and decisions that are made today. Therefore, if we have a goal of living a better life away from depression, it is better to focus on the present. This can be done by first focusing on today, having activities for the day, and when executing the activities, you should focus on the activity, and not the past or the future. This helps to improve reduce the worries of the future happening, and thus reduces the experience of negative emotions. It also relaxes the mind by letting it process little information. This does not mean that you are not in control of what will happen in the future, but you are building the future by concentrating on the present. Eat well today, interact well with those you meet, and just be happy about what happens within that day, wait for another day and do the same. Some people say, tomorrow may never come, because each day a new tomorrow comes; you are only certain about what happens today, and therefore make the best out of today and you will be happy.

# 29. The Change that Comes from Within

You're doing a wonderful job so far. You've already made a difference by making the decision to learn to master your emotions, understanding what they are, how they affect your lifestyle and what you can do to make a change for the better.

The next strategy is going to focus on how you can sidestep your emotional triggers by changing your emotions and using them to help you grow instead.

How to Change Your Emotions

Change is something that rarely ever comes easy. When you're trying to change what is part of your personality, the very thing that makes you human, and something that has been part of your life for so long, it's going to be even more of a challenge.

That's okay, because the best things in life are the things which are worth fighting and struggling for, and in this case, learning how to master your emotions is something you're going to fight for because it promises you a much better life.

A happier life, not just for you, but for the people you love. Emotional triggers will always be there because you don't exist in this world alone. You constantly have to interact with people, and even find yourself in situations that are less than ideal. It is bound to happen every now and then.

These factors are sometimes beyond your control, but there is something that you can control. You can control how you decide to respond. You can make a conscious effort to change your emotions, although it will take a lot of willpower to resist the urge to rise to the occasion and succumb to the temptation to react to what's provoking you.

It's going to be hard because you're going to have to go against your first instinctive response, to mindfully force yourself to react in a different way. A better way.

Changing your emotions may not be easy, but it is possible if you:

•Choose to Do Something That Makes You Happy

Those who struggle with their emotions are often unhappier than most, which makes it very hard to hold onto any kind of happiness.

When you're in a constant state of unhappiness, learning how to control anything becomes a challenge, let alone learning how to control something as powerful as your emotions.

Learning to master your emotions is not just about getting it under control; it is about reconnecting with yourself too and finding your happiness once more.

The best way to do that is to do something that makes you happy.

When you find yourself in an emotional situation and you're struggling to get a hold of yourself, walk away and choose instead to do something that makes you happy.

Each time you actively try to engage in an activity which brings you joy you'll find your negative emotions ebbing away quicker with each effort you make.

Harness the all-consuming power of happiness, because it's a good kind of emotion which will benefit you and everyone else around you.

A happier state of mind also makes it much easier for you to think with clarity, and in doing so, gives you a much better handle at controlling your emotions.

•Choose to Focus on The Solutions

Focus on the solution, not the problem.

The force of the emotions that we feel can still manage to get the better of us, even when we're trying hard to reel them in.

It is especially difficult because you're now trying to change the pattern of behavior that you have been used to for so long. The more you focus on the problem, the harder it is going to be to control your emotions, which is why you need to do the opposite.

Instead of focusing on the problems, turn your attention to the solution instead.

When emotions are running high, it is easy for someone else's anger, frustration or any other emotion they may be experiencing to rub off on you (emotions are contagious, remember?), and this will disrupt your own attempts at trying to master your emotions.

It helps to focus on the situation at hand to help you find a solution to the problem.

The challenge here would be trying not to lose sight of the real issue that you should be focusing on.

When faced with an emotional situation or person, remind yourself that there must be a reason for it, and you need to find out what that reason is before you can attempt to find a solution for it.

Instead of thinking "I'm so angry" or "I am furious", think about "What can I do to resolve this" instead.

There's always a reason and a trigger for every emotional outburst and getting to the root cause of it is how to try to resolve the problem.

•Choose Not to Follow the Crowd

When everyone else is feeling emotionally charged up, it's not going to help matters in any way if you join the crowd and add fuel to the fire.

Instead, try an alternative solution where you are the one who continues to remain calm instead. Allow yourself to be the one who keeps a cool head on their shoulders and take on the role of problem solver instead.

It's easy to let the emotions of others affect you, but the beauty of this situation is that you always have a choice, and you need to remember that.

If you choose not to follow the crowd, you're choosing to change your emotions. You now have the opportunity to provide that kind of solution for someone else.

•Choose A Time Out When You Need It

We all need a little space every now and then, especially when dealing with a highly emotional situation.

If you're the emotional one, don't hesitate to ask for a time out or a break if you need to remove yourself from the situation and take a few minutes to calm yourself down.

This is how you change your emotions, by choosing not to feed into it even more and taking a step back so you have a chance to breathe for a minute and try to calm your thoughts.

Emotions cloud your judgment and stop you from thinking straight, and you will be no good to anyone if you can't even think straight because you're too focused on how you're feeling to care about anything else.

The best thing you could do to provide a helpful solution would be to get some space if you feel like you need it. Recommend that they get some space too, so everyone can come back and revisit the issue when they're not as worked up emotionally and willing to listen to reason.

There are times and a place for effective communication and being emotional is neither the right time nor place. Take a time out if you need one.

•Choose Open and Welcoming Body Language Responses

Another challenging exercise in self-control and self-regulation is going to be making a conscious decision to remain calm, open and welcoming with your body language, despite the strong emotional situation you may find yourself in.

Adopt body language mannerisms which are inviting and you'll have a much better shot at getting your emotions under control quickly.

Body language is just as powerful as the words that you speak, and sometimes you could even end up making the situation worse without ever having said a word.

When someone is being emotional in front of you for example, and you roll your eyes and shake your head, you could end up aggravating the situation and making things worse, even if you never uttered a word the whole time.

As challenging as it may be, body language is just as important trying to resolve social problems which are caused by emotions.

What you need to do to change those emotions is to adopt open and welcoming body language gestures, which include making good eye contact, not crossing your arms in front of your chest, not frowning, clenching or muscles or display any visible indication that you may be feeling emotional yourself.

•Choose to Talk to Someone

We'll talk more about the negative effects of trying to suppress your emotions, but for now, one method of learning to keep your emotions under control is to talk to someone about it when it starts to feel like it might be too much.

Instead of keeping all those emotions bottled up inside you with no healthy means of release; choose instead to talk to a friend or family member with whom you're comfortable with.

Venting, as it is often referred to, can make you feel much better, almost like a weight has been lifted off your shoulders.

When that weight is gone, your head feels much clearer and changing your emotions then becomes easier.

Friends or family members who know you well enough might be able to provide some form of insight too and even give you their feedback which could prove to be useful advice.

Using Your Emotions to Grow

Your emotions can do one of two things.

They can either help you grow and become a better version of yourself, or it can hold you back and destroy your reputation.

The former open doors to new and greater opportunities, while the latter will leave you with a reputation that you're someone others should stay away from when you're unstable and emotional.

To achieve the former, you need to begin cultivating a positive environment for yourself, one that is going to make it easier to nurture these positive emotions and help you grow.

Here's the twist - it's not all about you. That's right, growing your emotions is not going to be an exercise that is entirely focused on you.

This time, you're going to be focused on making others around you feel good, which in turn helps you feel good.

Humans are social creatures by nature, and doesn't it always feel much better when you know you've done something that makes a positive difference in someone else's life other than yourself?

That's how you use your emotions to grow as a person. This is what you need to do:

•Be Appreciative

There is nothing that demotivates you and other people around you quicker than a lack of appreciation.

Showing a little gratitude and appreciation every now and then can go a long way towards turning your emotions around. When you're feeling terrible after a long day, just remembering that there's a lot in your life to be grateful for despite all that is enough to put a smile on your face.

Simple phrases like "thank you" or "nice job", maybe even a "we couldn't have done it without you" can make a real difference in your moral and that of others you spend your time with.

•You Need to Be Engaging

No matter whom you interact with, be engaging and go the extra mile to make a connection with them.

A genuine human connection is what we all long for deep down inside, and there's no one who is ever going to tell you that they enjoy being lonely.

No matter who you're engaging with, build a connection that is meaningful. With family, friends, and colleagues, out to them on a regular basis, congratulate them on little victories accomplished, and remember special moments like their birthdays and anniversaries.

These efforts will go a long way towards keeping the people who matter happy, and in turn, you will feel a lot happier too.

# 30. Remember to be Grateful

You must try and focus on the good things in your life instead of looking and dwelling on the negative things. Don't spend your time mulling over past failures in your life but instead look at the positive events that occurred in your life. Remember the important thing is that no one in this world is perfect and we all make mistakes in life but learning from your mistakes is part of life's journey. Don't beat yourself up over a mistake you have made in life but instead move forward and learn from it.

## Think of Others who are in Need:

Take time in your life to stop and give thought to others in the world that is in dire need of help. Many people in the world suffer terribly not knowing where or if they will have a meal each and every day. They have no proper homes, no clean drinking water many die each and every day from ailments that they didn't have to die from. If they only had food and clean drinking water to sustain them like you have. These are people that would gladly trade places with you who have a home, food and clean drinking water but yet you are still unhappy.

Sometimes it takes looking at what others do not have to realize how much you do have and how blessed you are to have the life you have. It may not be your perfect idea of a life but that is up to you to make choices that will improve the quality of your life. At least you have the freedom and options to make choices for yourself many do not have the freedoms you have.

## Stop Feeling Sorry for Yourself:

Instead of going on a self-pity trip perhaps you should instead try and focus on more positive things. When you feel yourself going into a depressive state where you think you are so hard done to stop and take a moment to think of all the people in the 3rd world countries that are dying of starvation each and every day while you sit feeling sorry for yourself.

Take this time and use it in a positive way such as making a donation to a charity either financial or by giving your time. You will feel much better than you would just lie around your home buried deep in a self-pity trip. You must get up and dust yourself off and begin taking actions in your life that will lead you to that happier life you seek but just remember to think about those who are less fortunate while doing so.

Show Compassion Towards Others:

Try and learn to have more compassion for those who may be homeless or in similar dire straits and think of ways that you can do your part to make the world a better place for all. Don't be afraid to go out into your community to find something that you may get involved with that is a good cause or group to join such as a religious based group.

Many religious groups help those in need; you could inquire what types of programs they may be involved in to help third world countries. Find a group or project that interests you in order to help others in need. You will get such a natural high from showing compassion and doing good things for those who are in great need of it.

## Remember to Tell Your Loved Ones You Love Them:

A good habit to get into that will not only make your loved ones feel better in hearing it but it will also boost your mood is tell them you love them. Don't take your loved ones for granted and just presume that they know that you love them, so you don't bother telling them. It is always nice to hear and reassuring when you hear a person say that they love you out loud. It helps to seal the bond with your loved ones keeping the relationships healthy by communicating clearly to others.

Don't cut yourself off from friends and family reach out to them for their support and you will get it. But you must be willing to let them know what is going on with you and try and talk about your feelings. Family counseling can be a good way to get some good advice on how to improve your relationships with loved ones. Try and be positive and give compliments to your loved ones not negative hurtful comments that can leave deep scars on a person's heart. If you have nothing good to say, then don't say anything. If you think positive thoughts, you should share them with others.

## Giving Thanks Daily:

There is so much in life that you should be thankful for each and every day; try and give thanks on some level each and every day. Point out things that others do for you to make your life better each and every day and make sure you acknowledge these things and give thanks to those that give them to you. If you are a religious person remember to give thanks to your higher power for giving you the life you live today. But just remember the power to improve your life lies in your hands; you must be the one to take the steps towards the healthier happier life no one can take these steps for you. Good luck in your journey to less worrying and more enjoying life to the fullest!

## How Is Worrying Related to Living?

Like loose motions, pimples and flat tires, worrying has plagued everyone at some point of time or other. Worrying could be defined as the excessive brooding over things a person does even before the mentioned things could prove to be a problem. It involves over thinking about issues that in most cases, aren't even worth it. Everyone goes through daily life crisis and strives through the day to solve them. The process involved requires thinking and mental application of the best possible ways to sort things out.

Worrying, however, is not all negative. It is a necessary process to anticipate and get prepared for an unforeseeable problem. Imagine not stocking up extra tires at the back of your car before heading out for a picnic to an uneven terrain. Worry beforehand about the possible circumstances so you don't end up in trouble later. Worrying is an unconscious part of the various ways in which humans have learnt to survive. It is Darwin's way to make sure humans don't adopt a laid-back attitude and be happy go lucky in life.

Worrying is a defense mechanism imbibed in humans to alert them of future issues. At times such issues are remote; while at other times these are imminent and deserve our special attention. It's the nature's way to put humans on their feet all the time. However, when practiced in abundance it can lead to health and life issues.

From being an alarm to be a stressful trait, worrying could change colors in minutes. It's that aspect of the human mind that keeps pushing for undivided attention to issues that don't deserve so much of mulling. Matters that could be solved by smart thinking and right decision-making skills complicate themselves when they fall into the cockpit of worrying.

Despite the urgency, some issues could be tackled in shorter and better ways. The more you think about them, the more monstrous they appear. Such equations turn devastating for you in the end. It meets no end when you spend more than the required energy in things that could be solved in other ways and methods.

One aspect of it says it's about eating, sleeping and existing like a creature on earth. Another evolved version says living is about having rights. Yet another definition argues that living is more than just survival. It's about being able to maximize your happiness and minimize your pains. Benthamanian school of thought would define living to be something similar. The reduction of pain and heightening of pleasure could be summed up to be living.

So, what do you think living is? Is it working dully at your cubicle and earning money by the month? Or is it preparing dishes for your kids and seeing them off to school? It could be traveling from one place to another, just for the fun of it. Like it's been mentioned before, living cannot be bound by limits and definitions.

For one person living could have an entirely different meaning than the next person. Though it differs from person to person, there are some aspects of it that never change and everyone, regardless of where they are and how they are, are entitled to some of such basic benefits of living.

One of the most vital aspects of living is enjoyment. You have the right to enjoy while living. Human wants never to cease. Be it in the form of a hobby or habit, wants never to stop expressing themselves. We seek wants because we aim for enjoyment. Now is enjoyment possible at all the times? There are times when full enjoyment is not possible.

Worrying interferes with life. It diverts your attention and allots to it such irrelevant stuff that you cease to live. People are often afraid of failing and that causes them to worry to such an extent that they stop living at all. Or they end up living so cautiously that they might as well not have lived at all.

It's no life to be worrying about money and relationships. Life's more than about petty things. Sure, money is what keeps you going, and relationships are necessary for one's romantic satisfaction, but those things are not all life has got to offer. Look beyond such limiting concepts and discover an entire new definition of what you've been calling life so far. Explore new dimensions to life and set out to redefine living. Stop over thinking and start learning how to. You have got a limited time on this planet; why not make every minute count? Why is it mandatory that you spend every moment solving, and not living?

# Conclusions

Many behaviors, such as losing weight, cannot be explained or even changed on the conscious, intellectual level. The key to success lies in resolving the mental imbalance so that those affected can find their inner balance and lose weight in a healthy way.

Eating disorders are often an expression of a mental imbalance. The lack of inner balance leads to blockages that prevent normal eating behavior. Practical tips and well-intentioned advice on losing weight are often ineffective because they only address awareness. Likewise, efforts made by those concerned to eat normally and lose weight associated with conscious effort often do not lead to success. Yes, sometimes these forced efforts to lose weight actually do the opposite.

Hypnosis is a temporary state of more acute concentration. It is a totally natural state of consciousness. We constantly pass in our life from one state of concentration to another. Therefore, hypnosis is totally familiar to us because of our daily experiences.

An effective and permanent change in eating behavior is most likely to succeed if the therapy starts at the subconscious level. So, the high success rate of hypnotherapy depends on losing weight together with the fact that it is possible to communicate directly with the subconscious. In hypnotherapy, the first step is to uncover the causes of obesity in the subconscious of a person.

Blockages that have manifested in the subconscious can be resolved in the hypnotic trance. By the way, no deep trance is required for this. A pleasantly relaxed, light state of trance is enough to work successfully. If the blockages acquired during childhood, adolescence or even in adulthood can be successfully resolved, the eating disorder can also be overcome so that you can lose weight on your wellbeing.

If you have been eating junk food all your life or been a chronic dieter your body needs to recover.

If you have never dieted and are thinking of going on a diet, I hope that this will have put you wise about the pitfalls and dangers. In short, don't go down the road of dieting, it is full of potholes.

This is why I feel qualified in writing this to help people have an insight into what it is like to be a recovered chronic dieter and bring to people's attention how politics can affect their attempts to be healthy.

This way of eating will be a transition!

An end to dieting, and then finding the best way of eating and the beginning of a healthy new you.

Make this a commitment for life and not just another diet. You can have the odd treat, and even a glass of red wine sometimes with your meal. But let the treat be just that, a treat! Not something that you are in the habit of doing all the time.

When you are eating out, ignore the jibes from friends. They will soon get used to your new and healthy way of eating, and may even follow you.

Use expressions such as "I don't eat that" rather than the disempowering "I can't eat that." This will let you keep your own power and not give it away to anybody else. "Don't" implies that YOU are in control. "Can't" implies that someone else's rules are controlling you.

Don't be afraid to ask the waiter or waitress for something different to accompany your steak. Ask for salad instead of chips. You will get so used to it that you won't think anything of it after a while.

Learn to cook. It is fun and you will be surprised at the concoctions that you can come up with using basic ingredients and adding spices and herbs.

## Changing your thinking

Changing the way that you think can make a huge difference in your weight management. There are beliefs that we all carry around with us from childhood. Many of them are necessary, such as cleaning your teeth because if you don't they will decay. Or wash your hands before eating and after using the bathroom, because of germs. These are just two very simple habits and beliefs. There are other more complicated ones that are passed down through families, or from parents to children, such as the type of manners we may have, or religious beliefs. But for now let's just keep it simple.

One belief that may be around is that if your parents were fat, so you will be too. You may have heard that this is genetic, or it's in the genes. But there is now a relatively new science known as epigenetics, and this is proving that although we may carry certain dispositions in our genes for illness or conditions, we can control the outcome with our environment. So because your parents were fat, does not mean that you have to be. You can change it by using a healthy way of eating and plenty of activity.

For example if someone dies of lung cancer and has been a heavy smoker, their offspring can lessen their chances of getting it by not smoking.

We also need to be aware of how we think in any given moment. One scenario often cited to me is people's work environment. I hear a lot about the struggle that office workers have when fellow colleagues insist on bringing in cakes for a birthday. The person who chooses not to include cake in their diet, often struggles with this, as they don't want to appear to be different and unsociable, or they feel left out.

Let's look at this a bit closer. There you are sitting at your desk and the doughnuts have arrived. Everyone is joining in and you have to make a choice.

I will cover briefly here something called resistance. There is a saying "What resists, persists" and this is true. Let's explore this a little further.

Imagine that it is the first time this has happened since you changed your way of eating, you can simply say "No thank you, I wish you a really happy day, but I am not eating that sort of food anymore". It is not a good idea to say that you are on a diet! That is like putting a red rag in front of a bull. Our society seems to hate people saying that they are on a diet. But the idea of watching our health is more appealing.

Be warned though, you will get some remark, but stick to your new principles. Because if you don't, then next time it will be even harder. Once they get the message the first time, as each time comes around, they will become familiar with the idea.

Another way to avoid the resistance though is to just accept the situation for what it is. Have just a little piece. But promise yourself that it will indeed be the one piece. That way there is nothing to resist. This will help you to become aware of your ability to make choices and changes. You are in control, and just because a certain food may have affected you in the past, you can change the story, and tell yourself that any weakness from the past, does not have to affect me now.

This can be quite a challenge for some people, and some life coaching or mentoring may be useful.

By this little exercise you will have learnt to change your thinking from "I'll just have one this time" to "I like eating this way and I am not going to let a moment's weakness or embarrassment spoil it"

Think about other occasions when we say, "No", and there does not seem to be a problem. Such as not having a drink because you are driving. On a parallel with that, isn't your health just as important and not having a cake because of it?

Using positive affirmations on a daily basis can be an incredibly persuasive method for attracting health, healing, and happiness into each day of your life.

Remember, as you start each day, it's up to you to decide if it's going to be a positive one.

Everyone has to cope with the onslaught of daily life, and tackle their own personal issues, in areas such as self-esteem, fears, and disappointments. However, by using positive affirmations, you can choose to approach life with a more positive attitude, be open to new opportunities, and expect good things to be attracted effortlessly into your world.

Throughout this, we've looked at what, why and how to use positive affirmations to gain personal strength, and to help us feel happy, healthy, and healed.

We've explored how to:

- Focus on what you really want.
- Use positive, uplifting, empowering words.
- Re-condition your subconscious, away from toxic thoughts.
- Understand why affirmations can fail.
- Identify the most beneficial affirmations for you.
- Correctly use the most effective techniques.
- Create believable statements that feel really good.
- Show gratitude for the positive changes in your life.
- Expect good things.

Positive affirmations, when used correctly, can offer a simple, fast and effective method for delivering long lasting change into your life. When you start to believe you are better, both physically and mentally, you will start to receive corresponding physical benefits to your health. When you feel more positive, you enable yourself to cope better with stress, to be more resilient to problems, and to fight off common ailments, thanks to an improved immune system.

Additionally, when you experience positive feelings, either through your engagement of affirmation techniques, or as a result of moving closer to your desired outcome, you will start to see more and more possibilities. As you experience greater levels of emotions, such as contentment, happiness, excitement, joy, and hope, you'll open yourself up to new opportunities, and ways in which you can experience even more of the positive things in life.

The conscious use of positive affirmations helps to bring about lasting, positive change by creating new affirming beliefs, deep in your subconscious.

The consistent use of positive affirmations can be a major component in letting go of negative beliefs. They can be used effectively to replace negative self-talk, which, when left unresolved, can have a detrimental effect on both our emotional and physical health, along with our ability to progress in any meaningful manner.

"Believing in negative thoughts is the single greatest obstruction to success."~ Charles F. Glassman

There are certain fundamental aspects you need to follow when you embark on a journey of affirmations. Get these right, and your personal affirmation statements will work amazing well:

| Trust | Know in your heart that they will work for you |
| --- | --- |
| Expectation | Expect a great outcome |
| Belief | Create believable personal statements |
| Power | Use your personal powers, and take action |
| Value | Be true to yourself and your purpose |
| Attention | Give intense focus to what you really want |
| Gratitude | Give daily thanks |

Pay attention to these hugely important aspects, as they help fuel the transformations you seek. Understand that each point above brings its own unique benefits, allowing you to continually attract more of what you want into your life.

The art of positive affirmation needs to be practiced, and honed, and practiced, to become a perfect fit for your own purposes.

Although affirmations do not necessarily offer a quick fix, they do offer a powerful solution to create positive, lasting change. The creation of well crafted, affirming personal statements, can help recondition our thoughts and beliefs, allowing us to feel good about ourselves in so many different ways. As they work deeply at the subconscious level to affect change in both your beliefs and attitudes, they can be a driving force for delivering change exactly where you want it.

Printed in Great Britain
by Amazon

46346717R00149